SOMATIC EXERCISES FOR WEIGHT LOSS (CHAIR YOGA)

A 28-Day Challenge to Burn Calories, Regain Body Shape, Reduce Belly Fats and Relief From Stress With Low Impact Workouts Done Within 10 Minutes

JOHN T. MUNOZ

Copyright Page

TABLE OF **CONTENTS**

INTRODUCTION

Somatic chair yoga offers a gentle yet effective approach to weight loss by combining mindful movement, breathwork, and body awareness while seated. Unlike traditional high-intensity workouts, somatic chair yoga focuses on engaging muscles, improving flexibility, and enhancing overall body awareness, making it accessible to individuals of all fitness levels and physical abilities.

Through a series of slow, deliberate movements and stretches, somatic chair yoga encourages participants to connect with their bodies, release tension, and cultivate mindfulness. By tuning into bodily sensations and breath patterns, practitioners develop a deeper understanding of their physical and emotional states, fostering a holistic approach to well-being.

Chair yoga provides support and stability, making it an ideal option for those with mobility issues or limited range of motion.

Additionally, the mindful aspect of somatic chair yoga promotes stress reduction and emotional balance, addressing underlying factors that may contribute to weight gain or difficulty losing weight.

Incorporating somatic chair yoga into a weight loss regimen can complement other forms of exercise and dietary changes by promoting body awareness, reducing stress-related eating, and improving overall physical and mental health. With consistent practice, individuals may experience improved posture, increased energy levels, and a greater sense of well-being, contributing to sustainable weight management and overall vitality.

BENEFITS OF SOMATIC CHAIR YOGA FOR WEIGHT LOSS

- Increased Body Awareness: Somatic chair yoga cultivates mindfulness and encourages participants to develop a deeper connection with their bodies. This heightened awareness helps individuals recognize hunger cues, emotional triggers for overeating, and areas of tension or discomfort that may hinder weight loss progress.

- Stress Reduction: Chair yoga incorporates breathwork and gentle movements to promote relaxation and reduce stress. By lowering cortisol levels and alleviating tension, somatic chair yoga helps individuals manage stress-related eating habits and make more mindful food choices, contributing to weight loss goals.

- Improved Mobility and Flexibility: Somatic chair yoga movements focus on gentle stretches and mobility exercises that help increase flexibility and range of motion. Enhanced mobility allows individuals to perform daily activities with greater ease and may encourage them to engage in more physical activity, supporting weight loss efforts.

- Enhanced Posture and Alignment: Practicing somatic chair yoga encourages proper alignment and improves posture by strengthening core muscles and promoting spinal alignment. Better posture not only reduces the risk of injury but also supports healthy digestion and boosts confidence, which can positively impact weight loss progress.

- Holistic Approach to Wellness: Somatic chair yoga addresses the mind-body connection by integrating physical movement with breath awareness and relaxation techniques. This holistic approach supports overall well-being by reducing emotional eating, promoting self-care, and fostering a positive relationship with one's body, which are essential components of successful weight loss and weight management.

Chair Cat-Cow Stretch

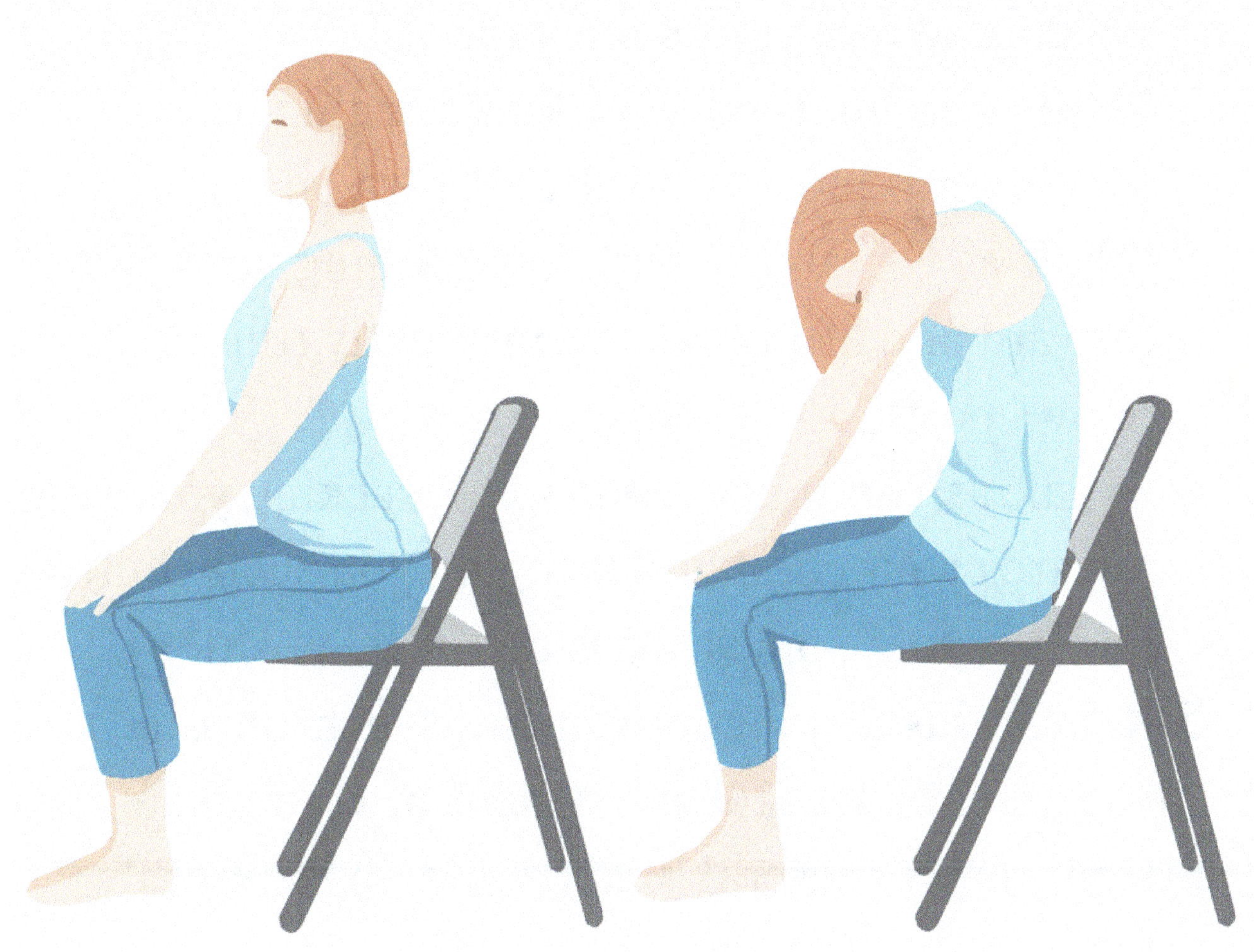

Chair Cat-Cow Stretch is a variation of the traditional Cat-Cow yoga pose, modified to be performed while seated in a chair. It's a gentle stretching exercise that helps to increase flexibility and mobility in the spine, shoulders, and hips, while also promoting relaxation and reducing tension.

INSTRUCTION

1. Sit comfortably on a chair with your feet flat on the ground and your spine tall.
2. Place your hands on your knees or thighs, whichever is more comfortable for you.
3. Inhale as you arch your back, pushing your chest forward and lifting your chin slightly (this is the "Cow" position).
4. Exhale as you round your spine, tucking your chin towards your chest and bringing your belly button towards your spine (this is the "Cat" position).
5. Repeat this flowing movement, synchronizing your breath with the movement of your spine.
6. Continue for several breaths, moving smoothly between the Cow and Cat positions.

MISTAKES TO AVOID

1. Always warm up before starting
2. Breathe Right
3. Perform the stretch slowly and with control to avoid injury.
4. Stay Within Limits

Chair Forward Bend

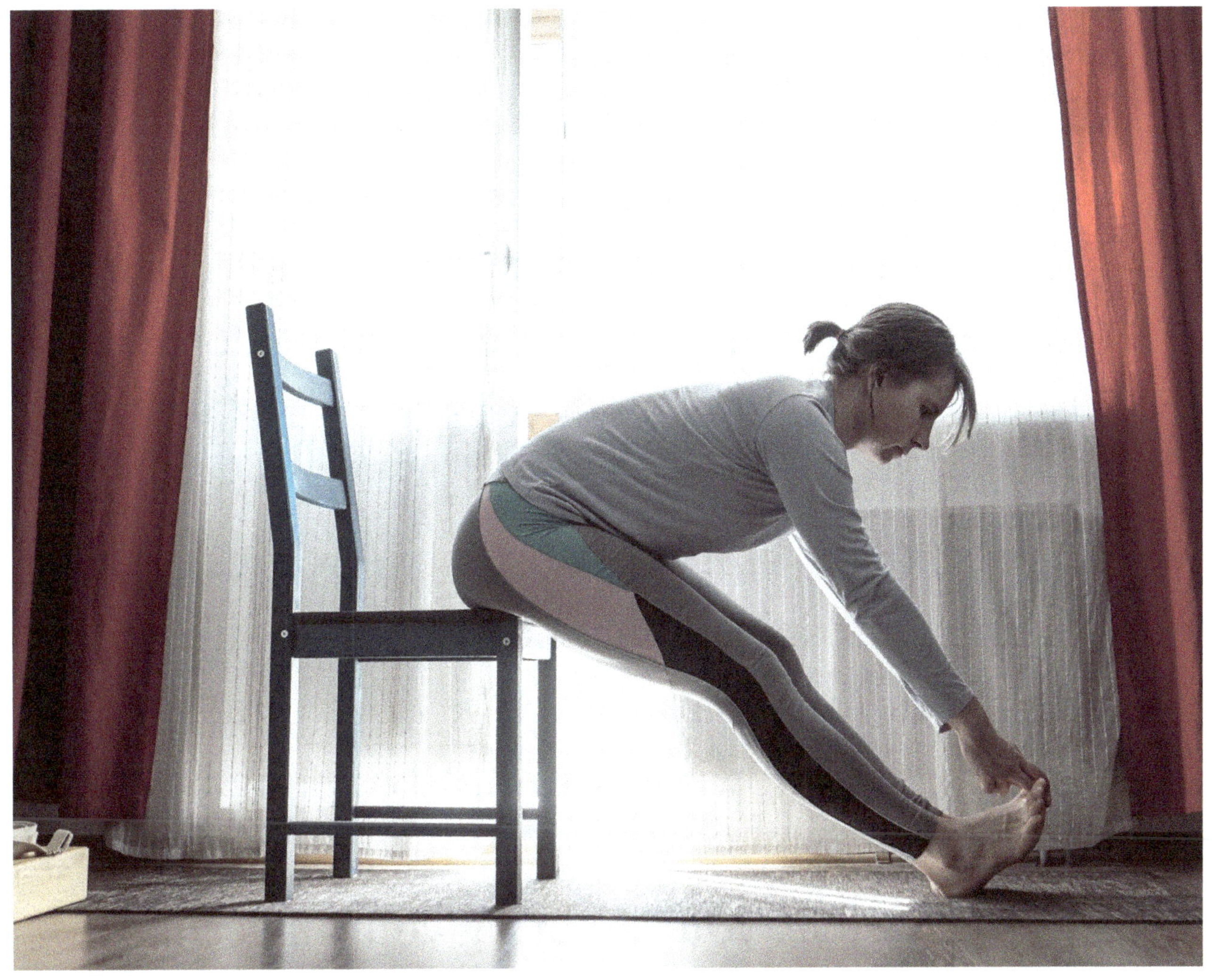

Chair Forward Bend is a yoga pose that combines the benefits of both Uttanasana (Standing Forward Bend) and Utkatasana (Chair Pose). It's also sometimes referred to as Chair Uttanasana. Chair Forward Bend helps to stretch the spine, hamstrings, and calves while also strengthening the thighs and core muscles.

INSTRUCTION

1. Begin standing with your feet hip-width apart, toes facing forward.
2. Inhale as you raise your arms overhead, palms facing each other.
3. Exhale as you bend your knees and lower your hips back as if you were about to sit in a chair.
4. Keep your weight back in your heels and your knees behind your toes.
5. As you exhale, hinge forward at your hips, keeping your spine long and your chest lifted.
6. Bring your torso parallel to the floor or as close as comfortable, allowing your head to hang between your arms.
7. If it's accessible, you can bring your fingertips to the floor or hold onto the sides of the chair for support.
8. Hold the pose for several breaths, relaxing into the stretch.
9. To come out of the pose, inhale as you press firmly into your feet, engage your core, and slowly rise back up to standing, lifting your torso.

MISTAKES TO AVOID

1. Avoid pushing beyond your comfortable limit
2. Don't rush
3. Don't overdo the Chair Forward Bend

Chair Spinal Twist

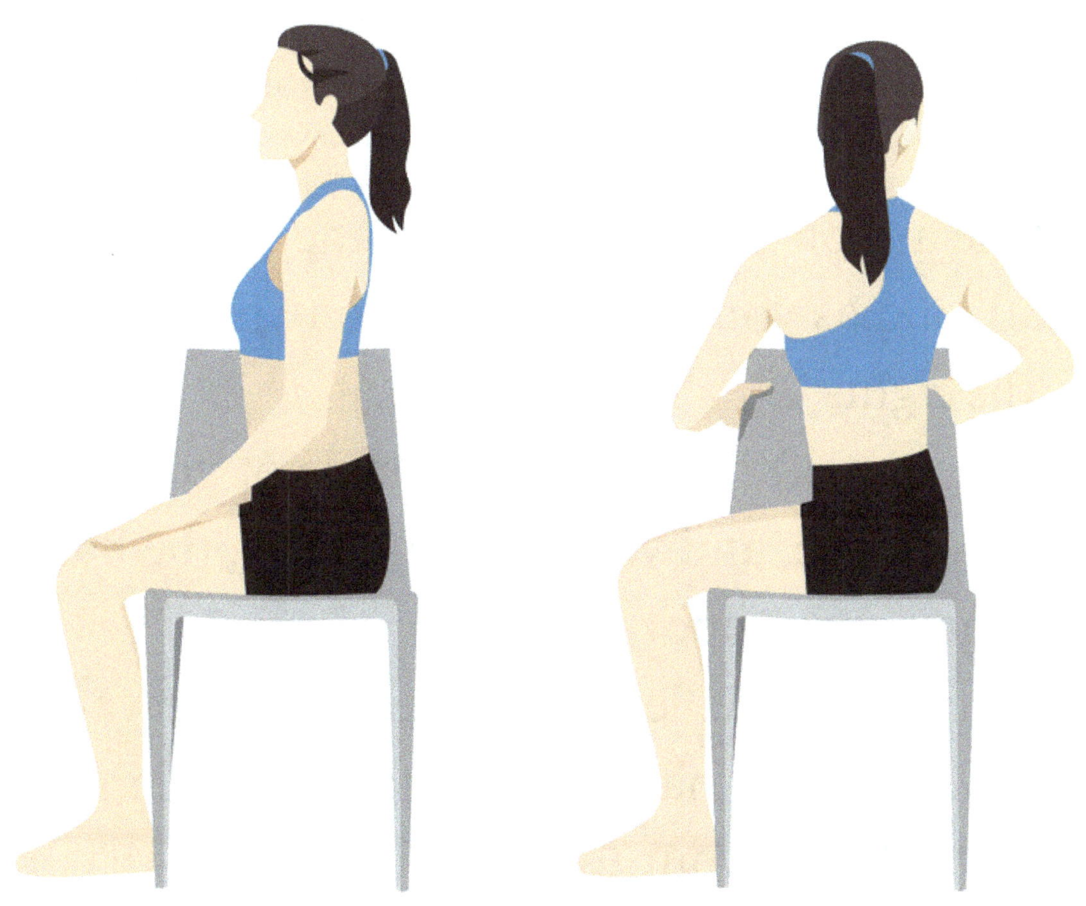

Chair Spinal Twist, also known as Seated Spinal Twist or Chair Twist, is a yoga pose designed to stretch and mobilize the spine while seated in a chair. It's a modified version of the traditional Spinal Twist pose, making it accessible to people who may have difficulty getting down onto the floor due to physical limitations or injuries.

INSTRUCTION

1. Sit tall in a sturdy chair with your feet flat on the floor, hip-width apart.
2. Keep your spine straight and your shoulders relaxed.
3. Inhale as you lengthen through the crown of your head, and as you exhale, begin to twist your torso to the right.
4. Place your left hand on the outside of your right thigh or knee, and your right hand on the back of the chair for support.
5. With each inhale, lengthen your spine upward, and with each exhale, deepen the twist slightly, gently rotating your torso to the right.
6. Keep your hips facing forward and your shoulders relaxed away from your ears.
7. Hold the twist for 30 seconds to 1 minute, breathing deeply and evenly.
8. To release, inhale as you slowly unwind the twist, returning to face forward.
9. Repeat on the other side by twisting to the left.

Chair Side Bend

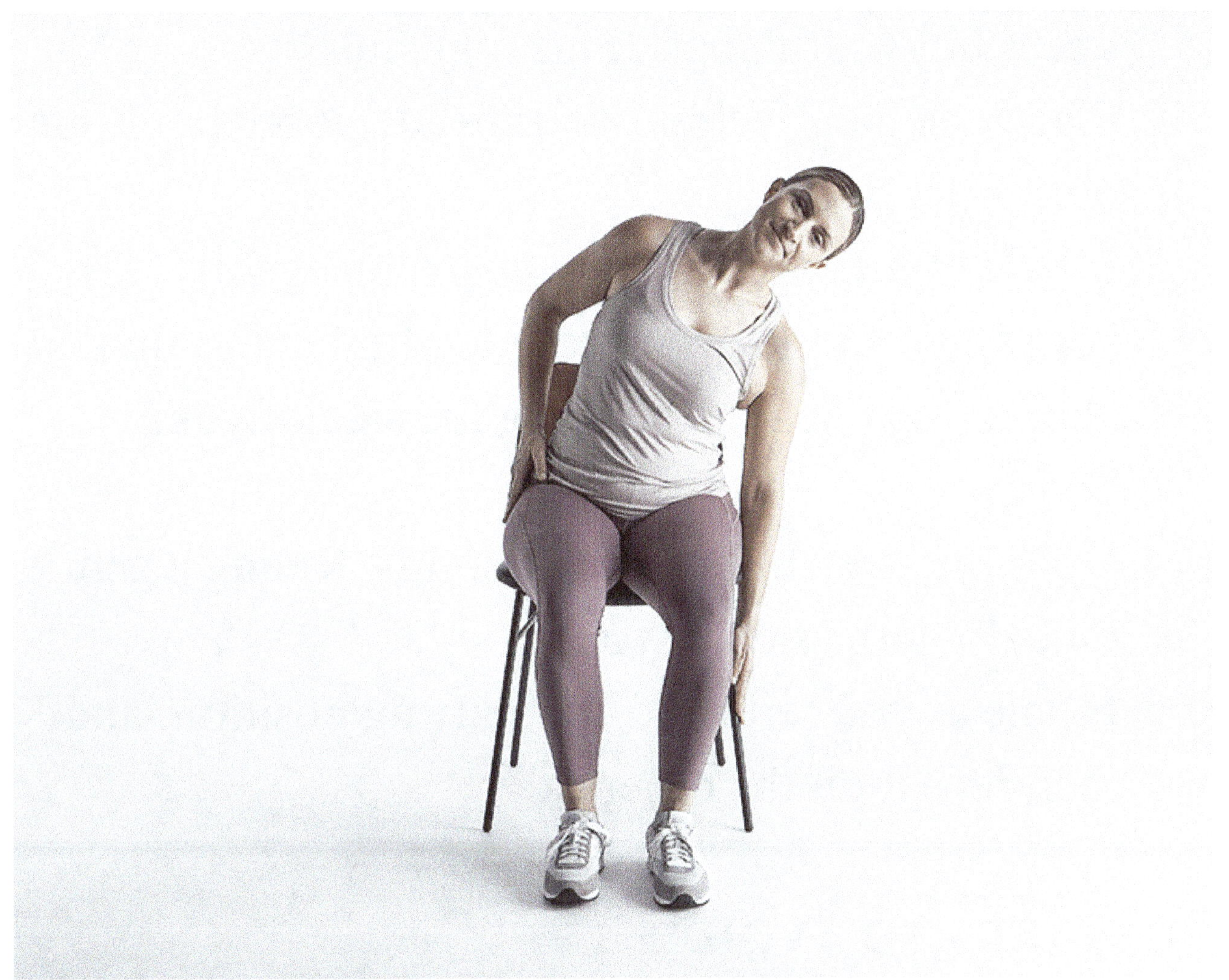

Chair side bend, also known as chair side bending, is a physical therapy exercise designed to stretch and strengthen the muscles of the torso, particularly the muscles along the sides of the body (the obliques) and the lower back (the erector spinae). Chair side bend can help improve flexibility, range of motion, and posture, as well as alleviate tension and discomfort in the muscles along the sides of the body and lower back.

INSTRUCTION

1. Sit on a chair with your feet flat on the ground, knees hip-width apart, and spine tall.
2. Place one hand behind your head, elbow pointing out to the side.
3. Inhale to prepare, and as you exhale, gently lean your torso to the opposite side of the hand that is behind your head, stretching the side of your body.
4. Hold the stretch for 15-30 seconds, feeling a gentle pull along the side of your body.
5. Inhale as you return to the starting position, and then repeat on the other side.

MISTAKES TO AVOID

1. Slow down to feel each movement fully.
2. Sit tall with feet flat to avoid strain.
3. Sync breath with each bend for relaxation.
4. Don't push too far; stay within comfort.
5. Always prep with gentle movements.

Chair Eagle Arms

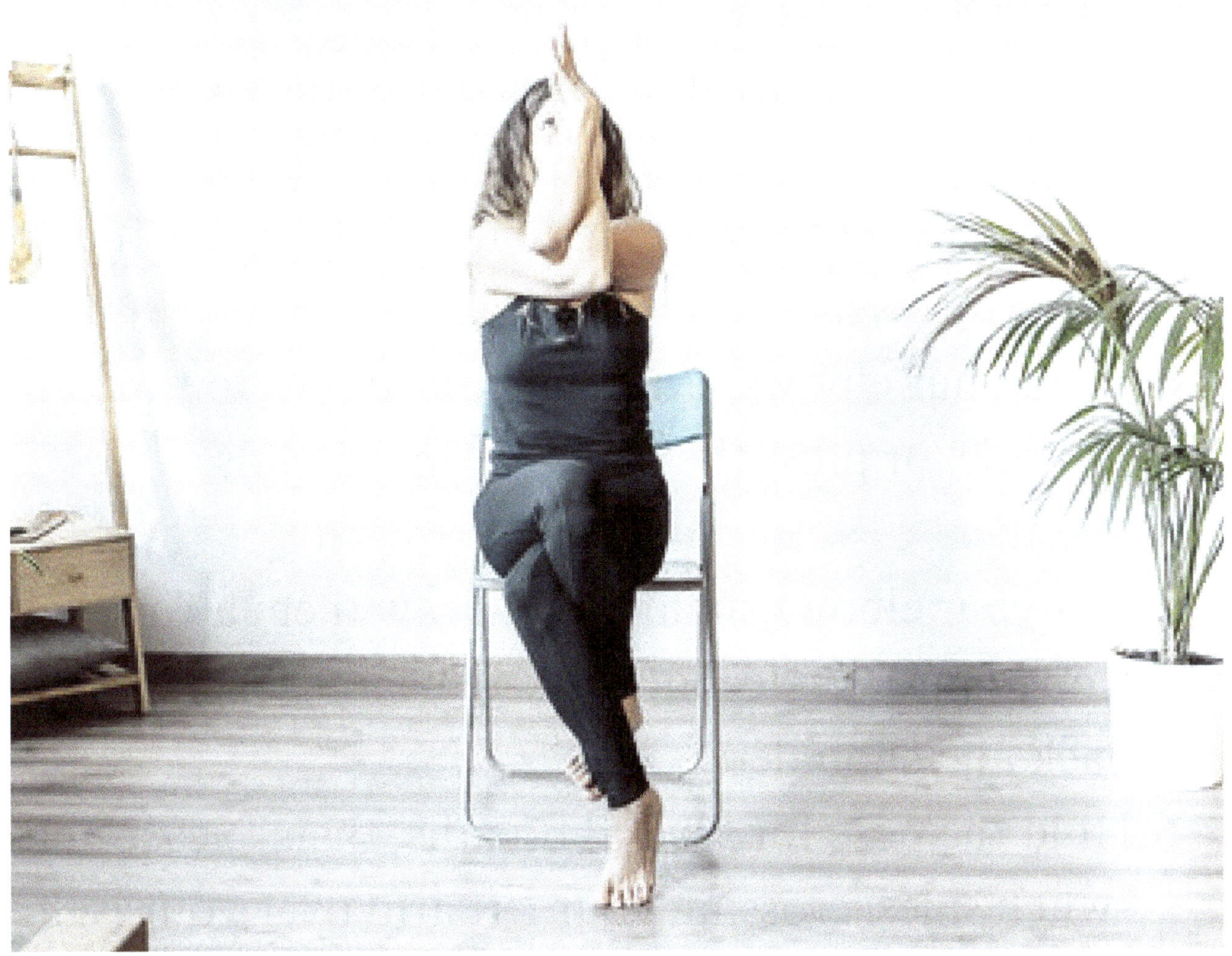

In yoga, the Eagle Arms pose involves crossing one arm under the other at the elbow and then twisting them around each other, similar to the position of an eagle's wings. It helps stretch and open the shoulders, upper back, and chest, promoting flexibility and relieving tension.

INSTRUCTION

1. Sit comfortably on a chair with your feet flat on the floor.
2. Inhale and extend your arms out to the sides, parallel to the floor.
3. Exhale and cross your right arm over your left arm at the elbows.
4. Bend your elbows, bringing your palms to touch if possible, or press the backs of your hands together.
5. Lift your elbows slightly and draw them away from your face, feeling a stretch across the upper back and shoulders.
6. Hold the pose for several breaths, then release and switch sides, crossing your left arm over your right arm.

MISTAKES TO AVOID

1. Slow down to feel the stretch fully and prevent strain.
2. Sync breath with movement for relaxation.
3. Avoid overextending arms or hunching shoulders.
4. Prep with gentle stretches to enhance effectiveness.

Chair Shoulder Opener

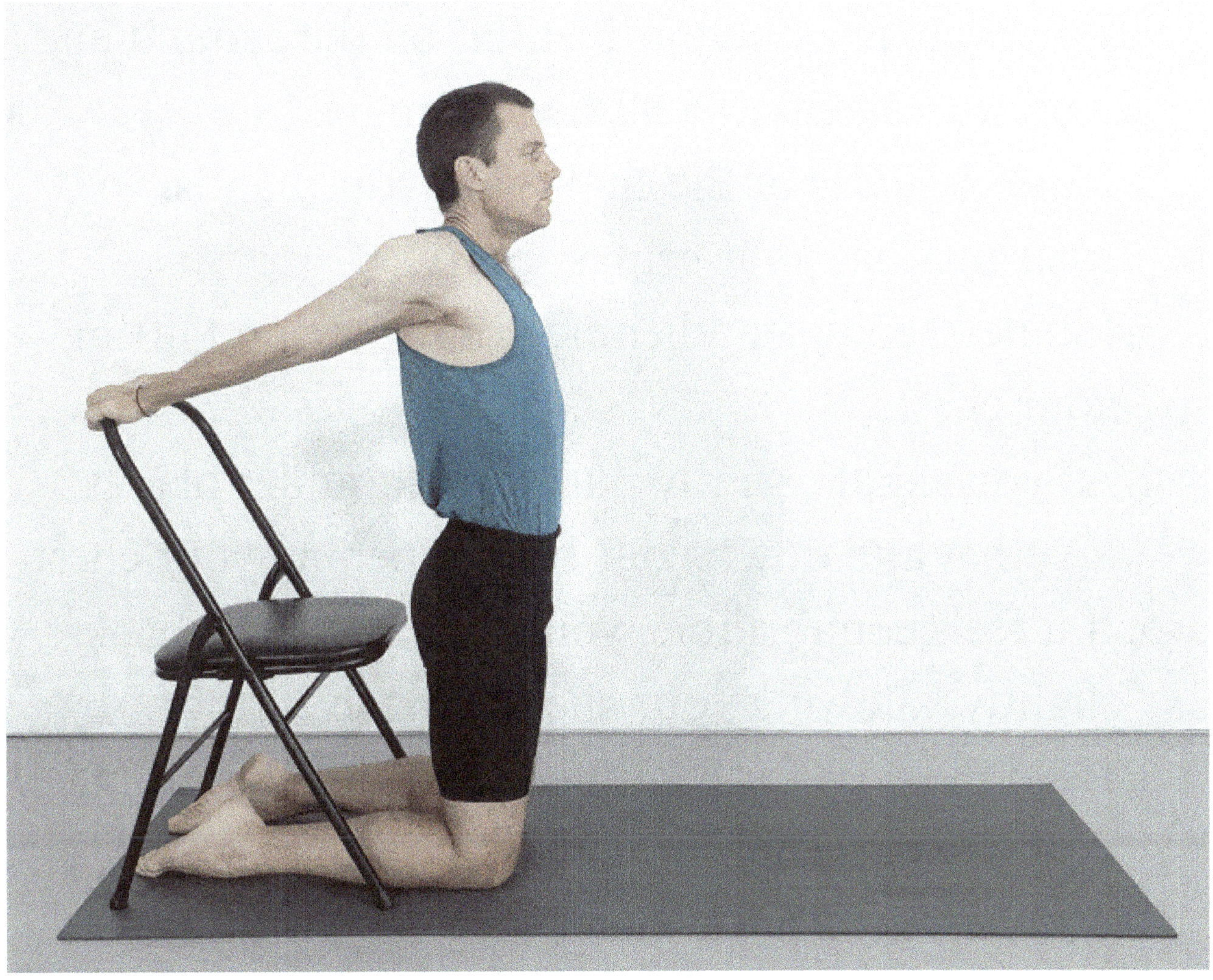

The Chair Shoulder Opener is a yoga pose that helps stretch and open up the shoulders, chest, and upper back. This stretch can help relieve tension in the shoulders and upper back, improve posture, and increase flexibility in the chest muscles.

INSTRUCTION

1. Begin by sitting comfortably on the edge of a sturdy chair with your feet flat on the ground and your knees bent at a 90-degree angle.
2. Hold the sides of the chair with your hands, ensuring that your grip is secure.
3. Inhale deeply, lengthening your spine and lifting your chest.
4. As you exhale, gently pull your shoulder blades together and down your back, opening your chest.
5. If it feels comfortable, you can gently lean back slightly, allowing your chest to open further.
6. Hold the pose for 20-30 seconds while breathing deeply and evenly.
7. To release the pose, inhale and slowly return to an upright position.

MISTAKES TO AVOID

1. Always listen to the body.
2. Sync breath with movement for relaxation.
3. Avoid overextending arms or hunching shoulders.
4. Prep with gentle stretches to enhance effectiveness.

Chair Mountain Pose

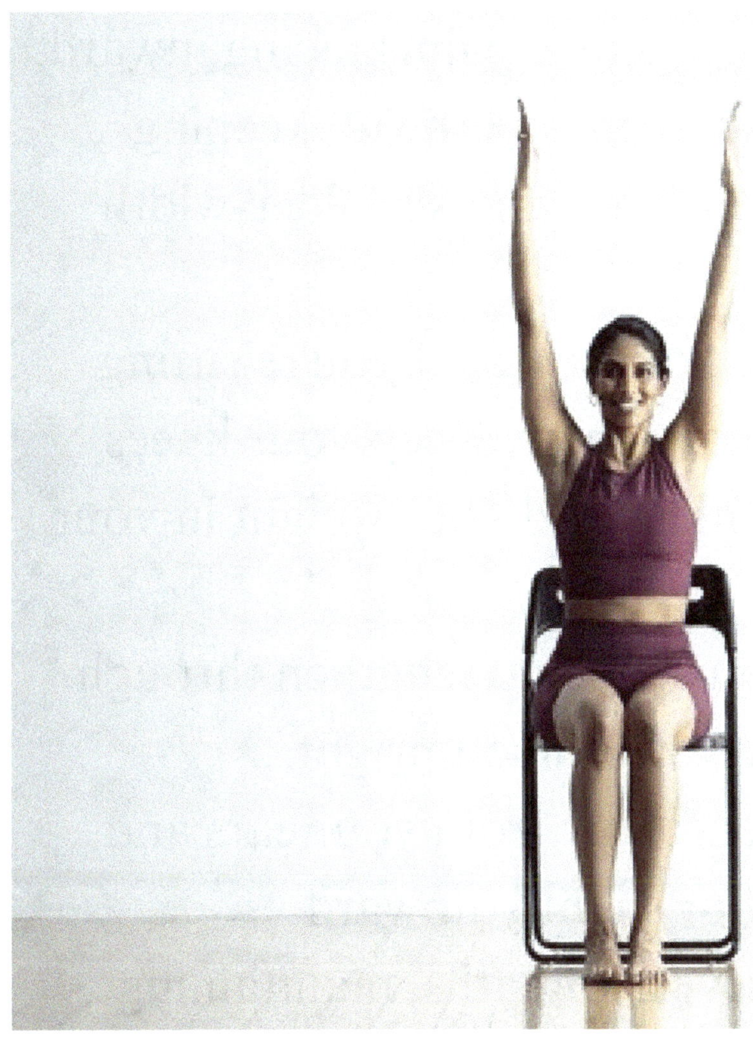

Chair Mountain Pose, also known as Utkatasana in Sanskrit, is a standing yoga pose that combines the strength-building benefits of a squat with the stretching and lengthening benefits of a forward bend. It strengthens the thighs, calves, and ankles, while also stretching the shoulders and chest. It can help improve balance, posture, and core strength.

INSTRUCTION

1. Begin standing tall with your feet hip-width apart and your arms at your sides, palms facing inward.
2. Inhale and raise your arms overhead, keeping them parallel to each other and shoulder-width apart.
3. Exhale and bend your knees, as if you're sitting back into an imaginary chair. Keep your knees aligned with your ankles and your weight in your heels.
4. Engage your core muscles and lengthen through your spine, keeping your torso upright.
5. Relax your shoulders away from your ears and gaze straight ahead or slightly upward.
6. Hold the pose for several breaths, maintaining steady breathing.
7. To release, inhale and straighten your legs, lifting your arms overhead. Exhale as you lower your arms back to your sides.

MISTAKES TO AVOID

1. Always listen to the body.
2. Sync breath with movement
3. Avoid excessive arching or rounding to prevent strain.

Chair Raised Hands Pose

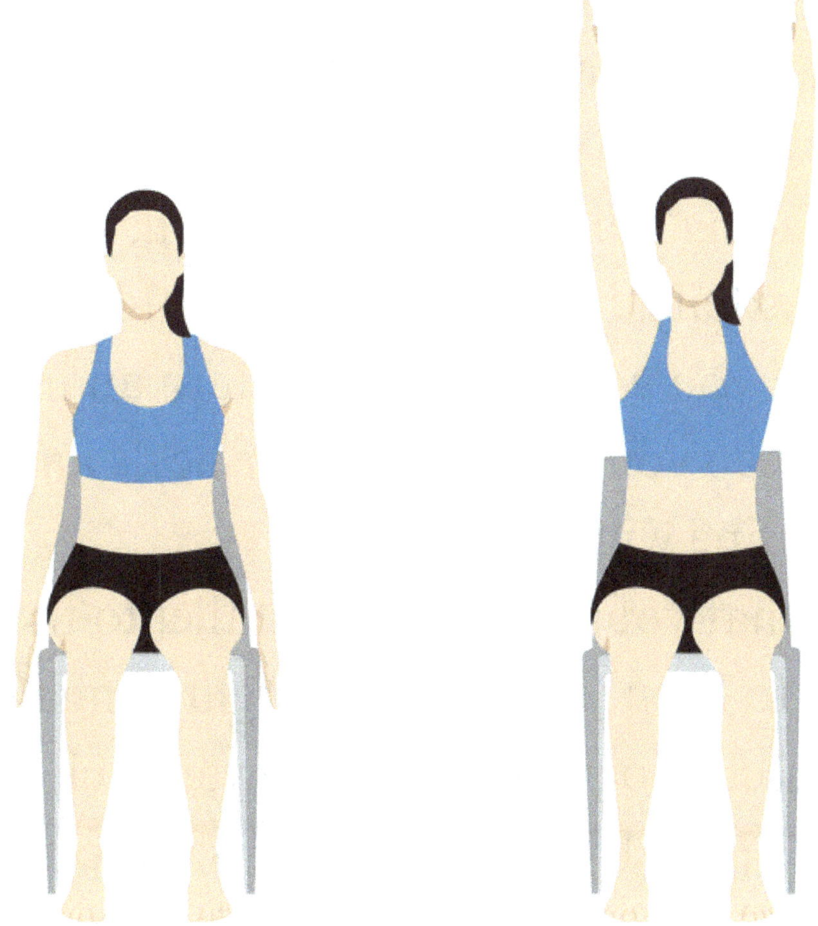

Chair Raised Hands Pose" is a yoga pose that combines elements of both Chair Pose (Utkatasana) and Raised Hands Pose (Urdhva Hastasana). Thus pose strengthens the legs, opens the chest, and improves posture. It also helps to build focus and concentration.

INSTRUCTION

1. Begin by standing tall in Mountain Pose (Tadasana) at the front of your mat, with your feet hip-width apart and your arms by your sides.
2. Inhale deeply as you raise your arms overhead, palms facing each other or touching.
3. As you exhale, bend your knees and lower your hips as if you were sitting back into an imaginary chair. Keep your weight in your heels and your knees in line with your ankles.
4. Ensure that your thighs are parallel to the floor, and try to keep your torso upright. Engage your core muscles to protect your lower back.
5. Hold the pose for several breaths, keeping your arms raised overhead. You can deepen the stretch by reaching your fingertips toward the ceiling.
6. To release the pose, straighten your legs and lower your arms back down to your sides as you exhale.

MISTAKES TO AVOID

1. Ignoring Warm-Up
2. Overextending
3. Neglecting Breathing

Chair Warrior I

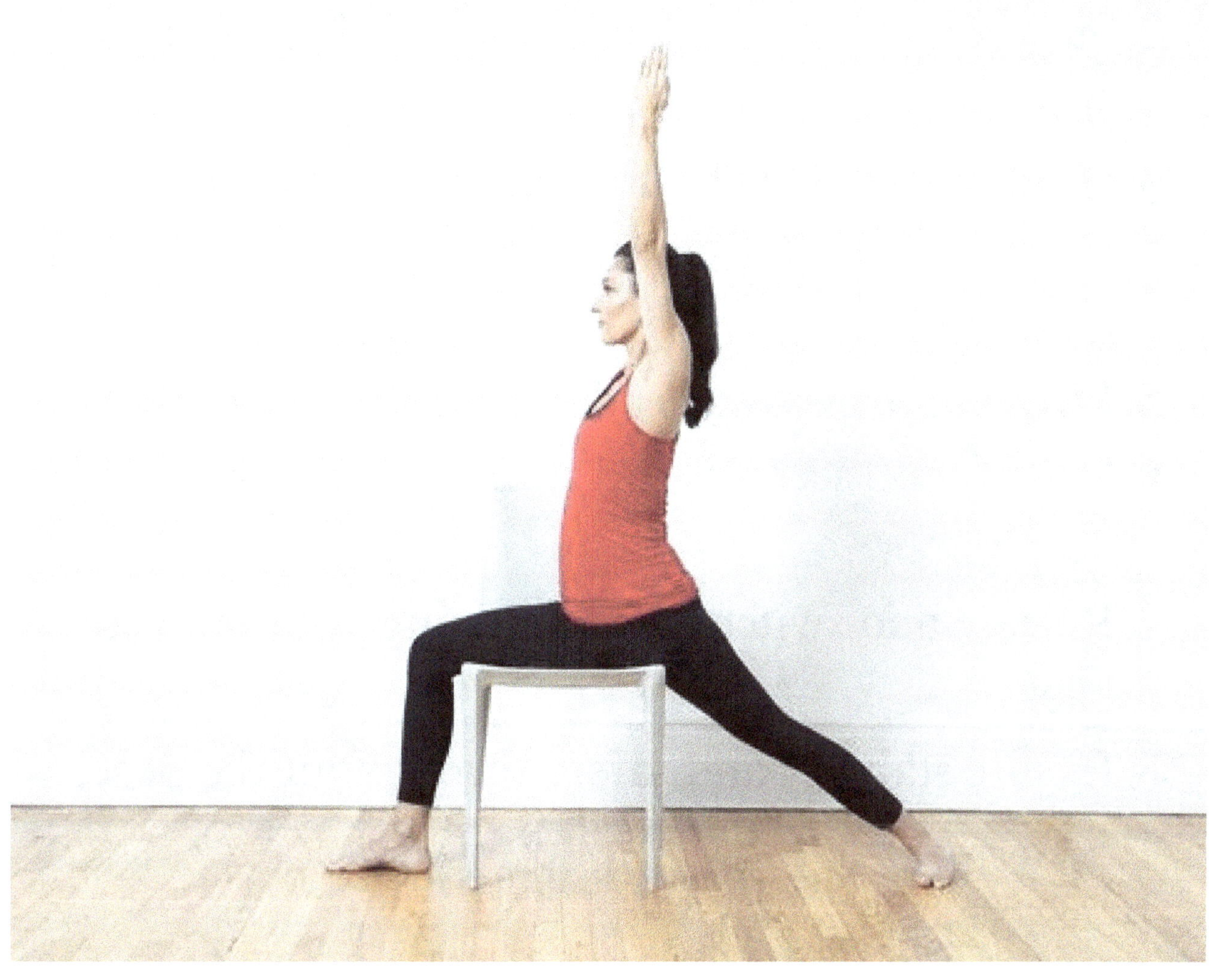

Chair Warrior I is a variation of the traditional Warrior I yoga pose that utilizes a chair for support and stability. Chair Warrior I is a great modification for those who may have difficulty with balance or mobility issues.

INSTRUCTION

1. Stand facing a chair with feet hip-width apart.
2. Step your right foot back, about 2-3 feet behind you.
3. Hold onto the back of the chair for support.
4. Bend your left knee into a lunge, keeping the right leg straight.
5. Lift your arms overhead, parallel to each other.
6. Hold for 30 seconds to 1 minute while breathing deeply.
7. Release and switch sides, stepping your left foot back.
8. Ensure stability and safety throughout the pose.

MISTAKES TO AVOID

1. Ignoring Warm-Up
2. Overextending
3. Avoid arching

Chair Warrior II

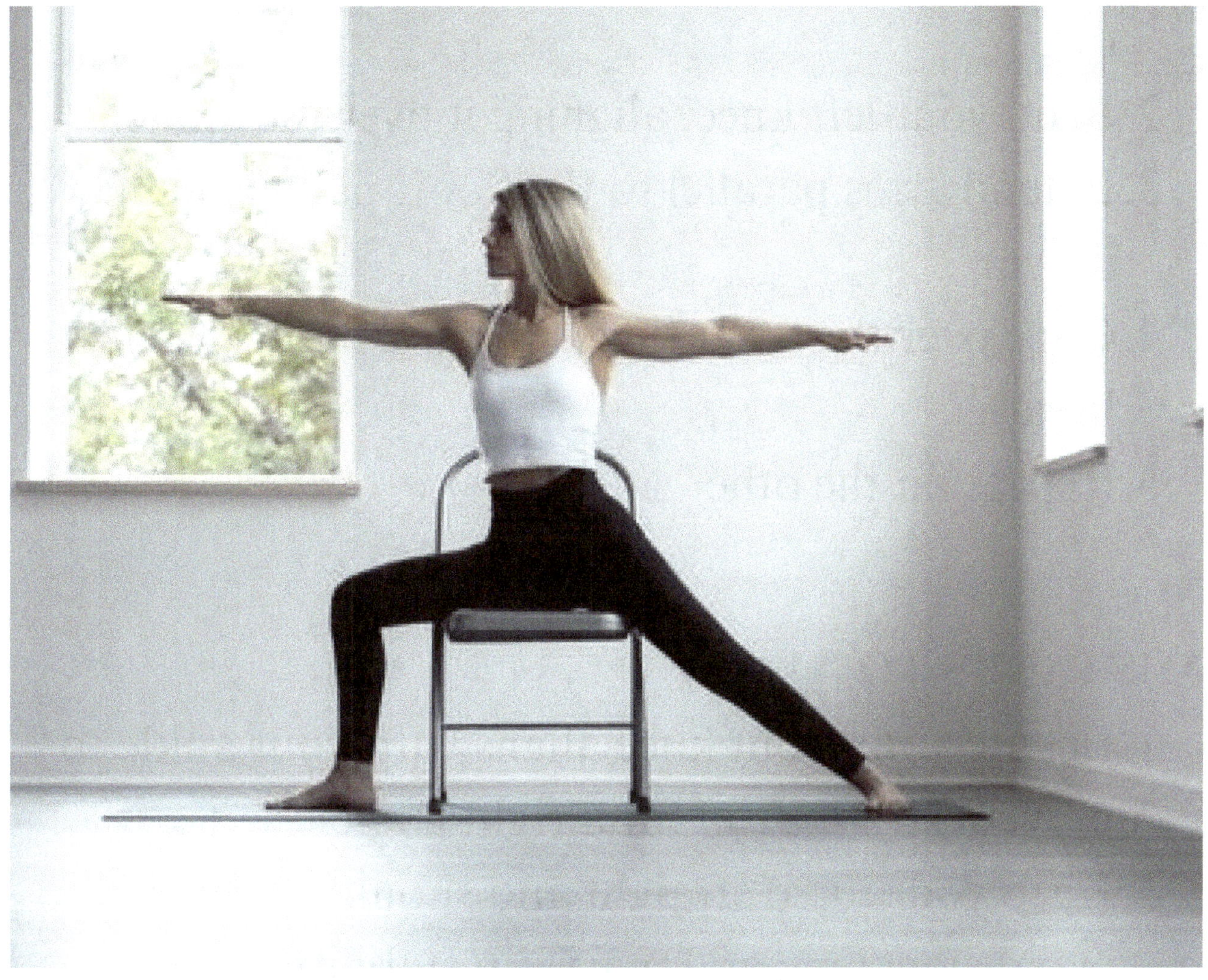

Warrior Pose Ii Chair (Virabhadrasana Ii Chair) is a supported variation of the foundational pose, Warrior Pose Ii. The difference is that the lower body is supported on a chair, taking the weight or pressure off the knee and ankle joints.

INSTRUCTION

1. Sit tall, extend your right leg back and turn toes out.
2. Bend your left knee, aligning it over the ankle.
3. Extend arms parallel to the floor, palms facing down.
4. Gaze over the front fingertips and hold for a few breaths.
5. Repeat on the other side.

MISTAKES TO AVOID

1. Ensure your front knee aligns with your ankle to prevent strain. Aim for a right angle.
2. Keep your torso straight and shoulders relaxed to avoid slouching and maintain stability.
3. Avoid excessive arching of your lower back by engaging your core and keeping your tailbone slightly tucked.
4. Maintain a steady breath flow to stay relaxed and focused during the pose, inhaling and exhaling deeply.

Chair Warrior III

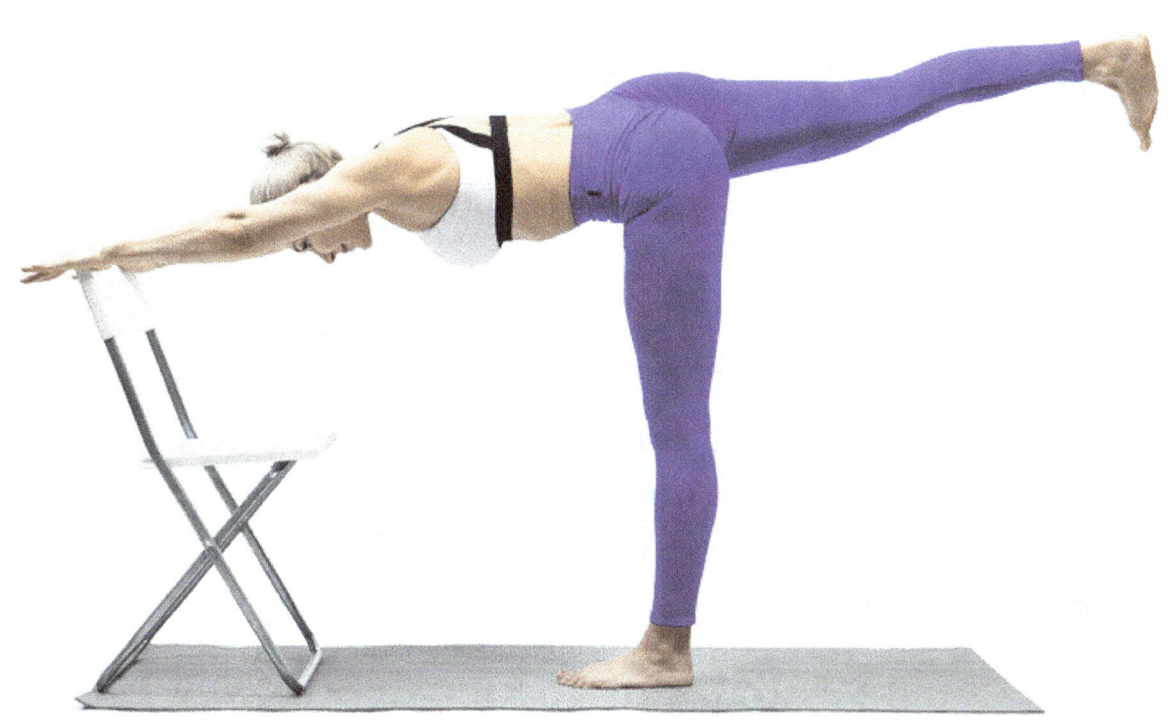

 Warrior III (Virabhadrasana III) is a balancing pose that strengthens the legs and core, improves focus, and enhances stability.

INSTRUCTION

1. Sit tall, extend your right leg back, and lean forward.
2. Keep hips square and reach arms forward or alongside the body.
3. Engage your core and hold for a few breaths.
4. Repeat on the other side.

MISTAKES TO AVOID

1. Keep your spine straight and shoulders relaxed.
2. Ensure your hips and shoulders stay level.
3. Avoid locking your standing knee.
4. Keep shoulders relaxed, away from ears.
5. Maintain a straight line from extended leg to torso.

Chair High Lunge

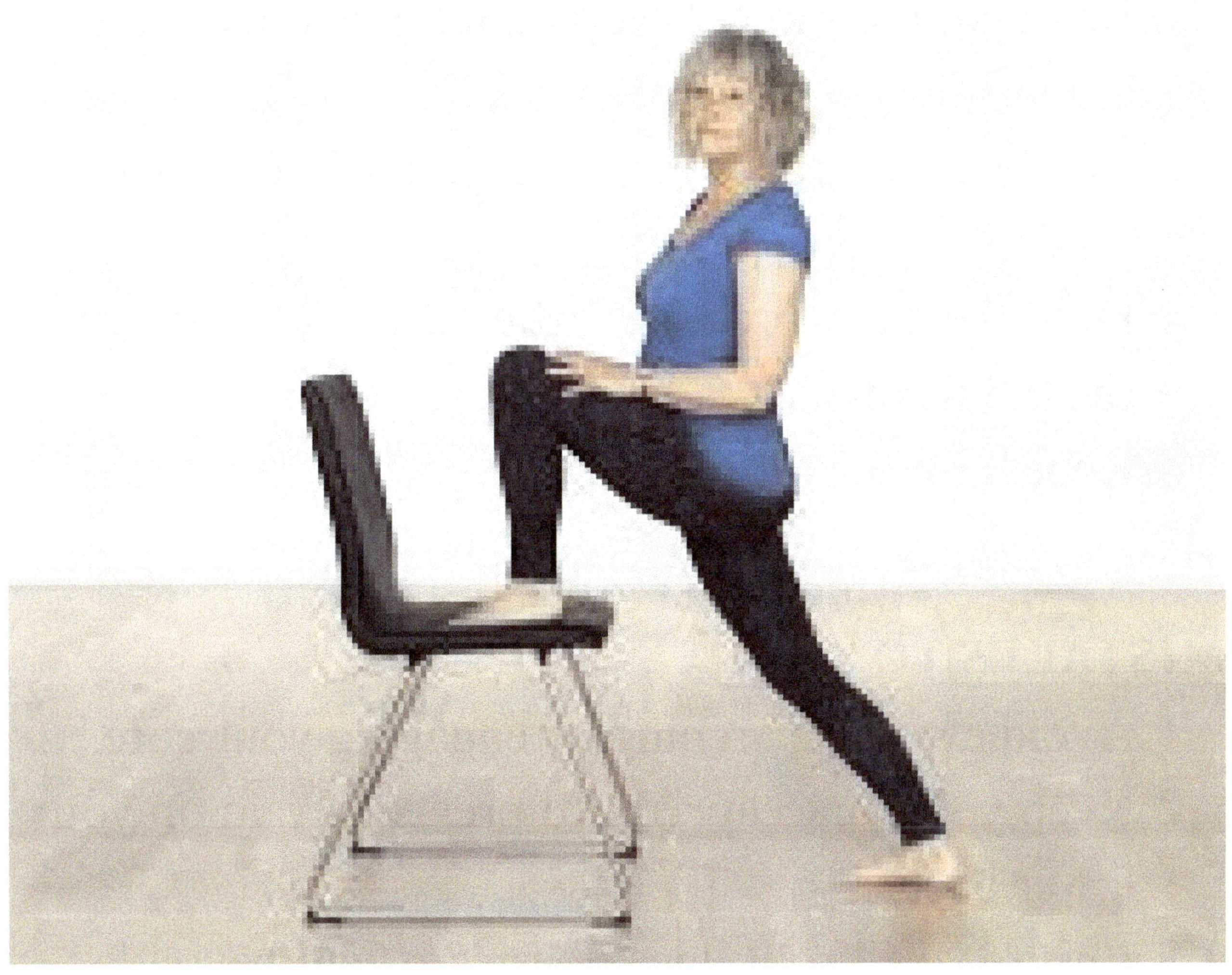

Chair High Lunge" is a yoga pose that combines elements of both Chair Pose (Utkatasana) and High Lunge (Ashta Chandrasana). Chair High Lunge combines the strengthening and grounding benefits of Chair Pose with the hip-opening and stretching benefits of High Lunge.

INSTRUCTION

1. Sit tall, extend your right leg back.
2. Bend your left knee, keeping it aligned over the ankle.
3. Inhale, raise arms overhead, palms facing each other.
4. Hold for a few breaths, feeling a stretch through the hip flexors.
5. Repeat on the other side.

MISTAKES TO AVOID

1. Avoid excessive arching by engaging your core.
2. Keep your torso upright to prevent strain on your lower back.
3. Ensure your front knee doesn't extend beyond your ankle to avoid potential strain.
4. Maintain a firm foundation with your back foot to prevent wobbling.
5. Remember to breathe steadily to oxygenate muscles and promote relaxation.

Chair Boat Pose (Navasana)

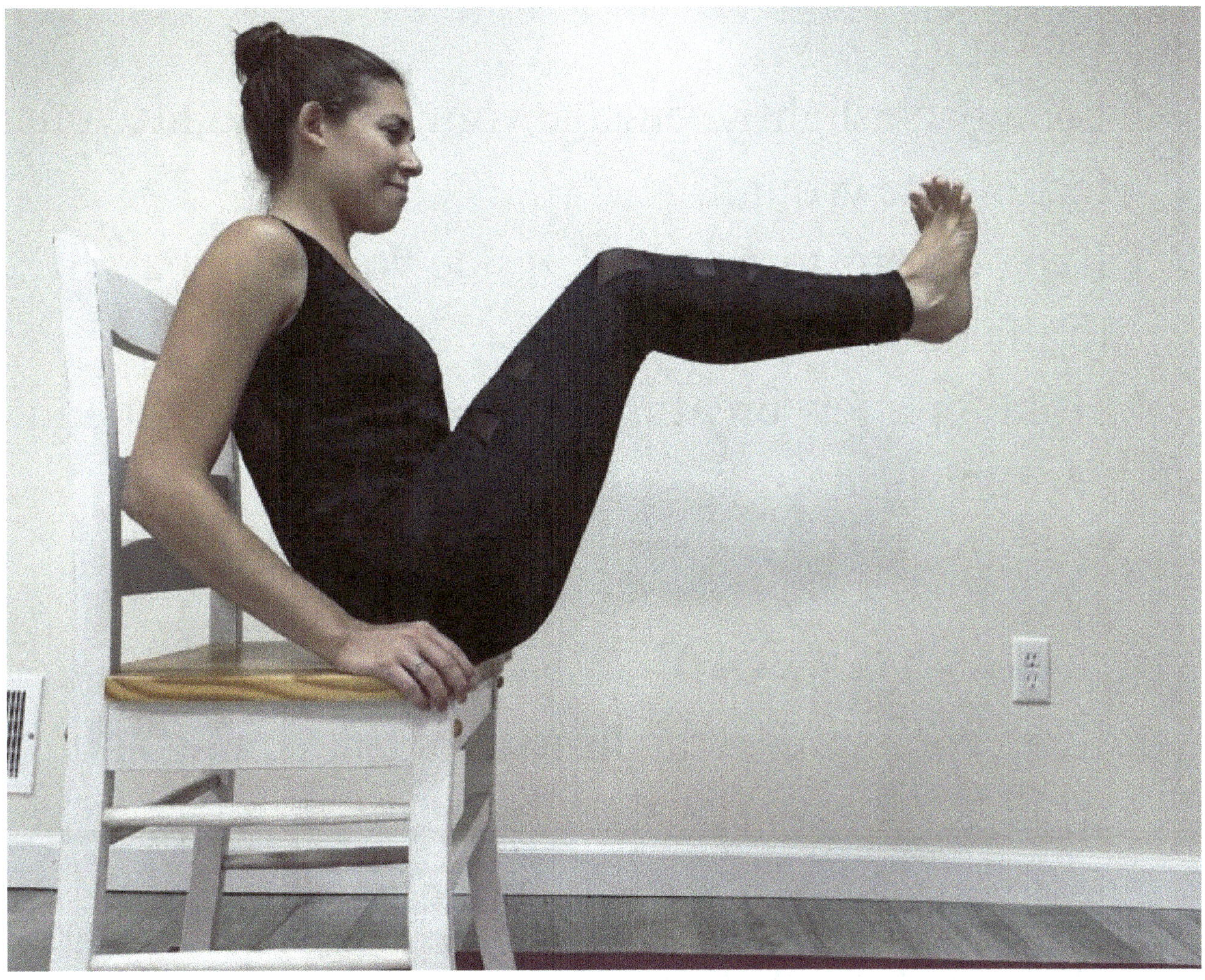

Chair Boat Pose, also known as Navasana in Sanskrit, is a yoga posture that combines elements of both sitting and balancing. It is an excellent posture for strengthening the core muscles, including the abdominals, hip flexors, and lower back. It also helps improve balance, concentration, and overall body awareness.

INSTRUCTION

1. Sit toward the front edge of the chair, feet flat on the floor.
2. Lean back slightly, engage your core, and lift your feet off the ground.
3. Extend arms forward alongside your legs, parallel to the floor.
4. Hold for a few breaths, keeping spine straight and core engaged.

MISTAKES TO AVOID

1. Keep your spine straight to avoid slouching and strain.
2. Lift your chest to prevent rounding of the back and maintain openness.
3. Keep legs lifted parallel to the ground to engage core muscles fully.
4. Relax your toes instead of clenching them to prevent unnecessary tension.
5. Remember to breathe steadily to stay relaxed and focused.

Chair Tree Pose (Vrksasana)

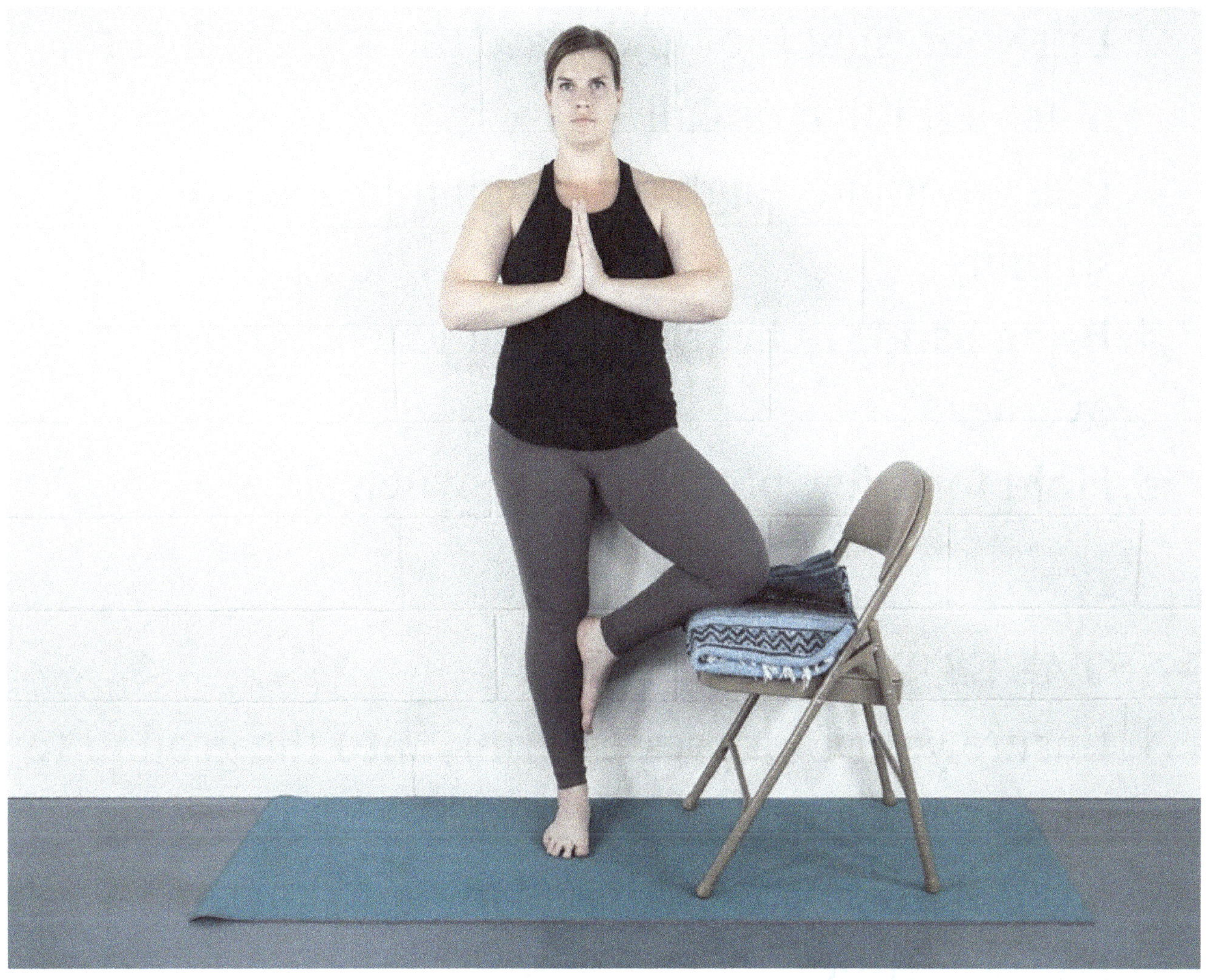

Chair Tree Pose, also known as "Vrksasana" in Sanskrit, is a variation of the traditional Tree Pose (Vrksasana) in yoga. In this variation, the practitioner combines the stability and grounding of Chair Pose (Utkatasana) with the balance and focus of Tree Pose.

INSTRUCTION

1. Sit tall with feet flat on the floor.
2. Lift your right foot and place the sole against the inner left thigh or calf.
3. Press foot into thigh and thigh into foot for stability.
4. Bring hands to heart center or extend arms overhead.
5. Hold for a few breaths, then switch sides.

MISTAKES TO AVOID

1. Ensure your foot presses firmly into the ground to avoid wobbling.
2. Keep shoulders relaxed and away from ears to prevent tension.
3. Engage your core muscles to maintain balance and stability.
4. Avoid placing your foot too high on the opposite leg to prevent strain on the knee.
5. Keep your gaze soft and steady to aid in balance without straining the neck.

Chair Raised Leg Pose

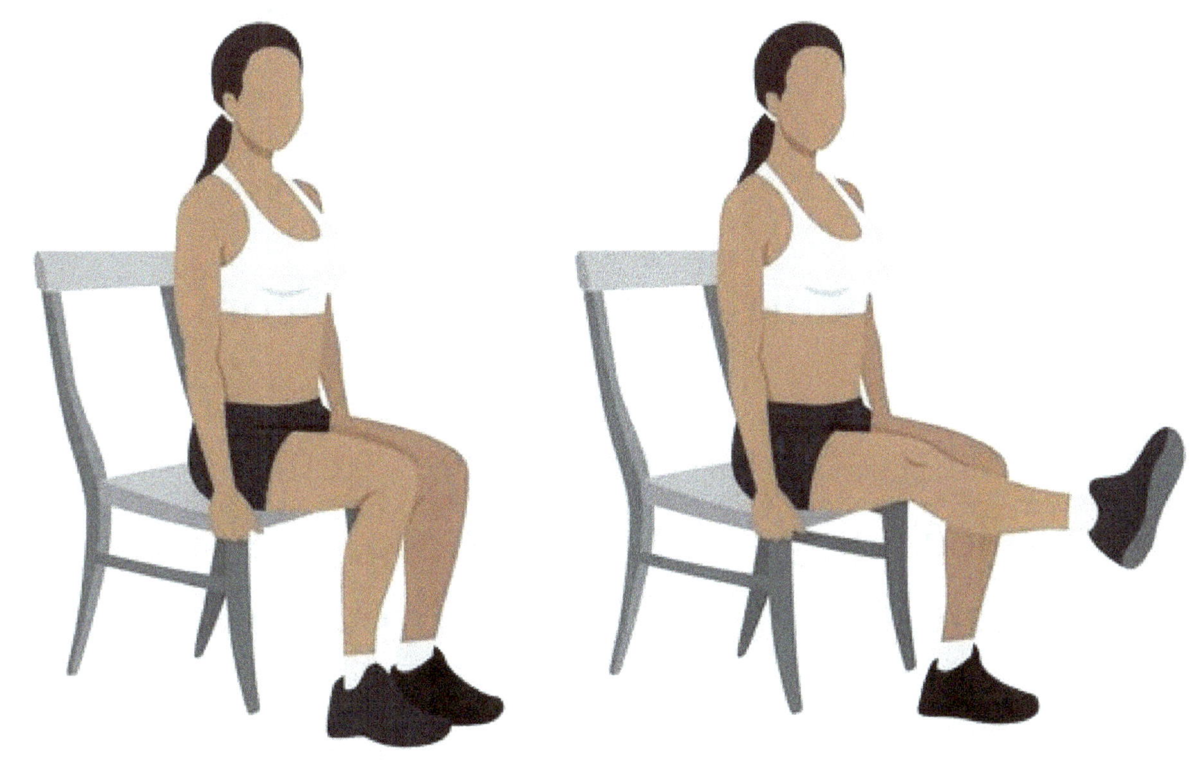

Chair Raised Leg Pose, also known as Utkatasana (OOT-kah-TAHS-uh-nuh) in Sanskrit, is a variation of the traditional Chair Pose (Utkatasana). In this pose, one leg is lifted off the ground while maintaining the posture of the Chair Pose with the other leg.

INSTRUCTION

1. Sit tall with legs extended.
2. Inhale, lift one leg off the floor, keeping it straight.
3. Hold for a few breaths, engaging the quadriceps.
4. Repeat with the other leg.

MISTAKES TO AVOID

1. Maintain a stable spine and engaged core.
2. Keep shoulders down to avoid tension.
3. Ensure hips stay parallel to the ground.
4. Avoid locking your standing knee.
5. Keep extended leg aligned with your torso.

Chair Knee to Chest Pose

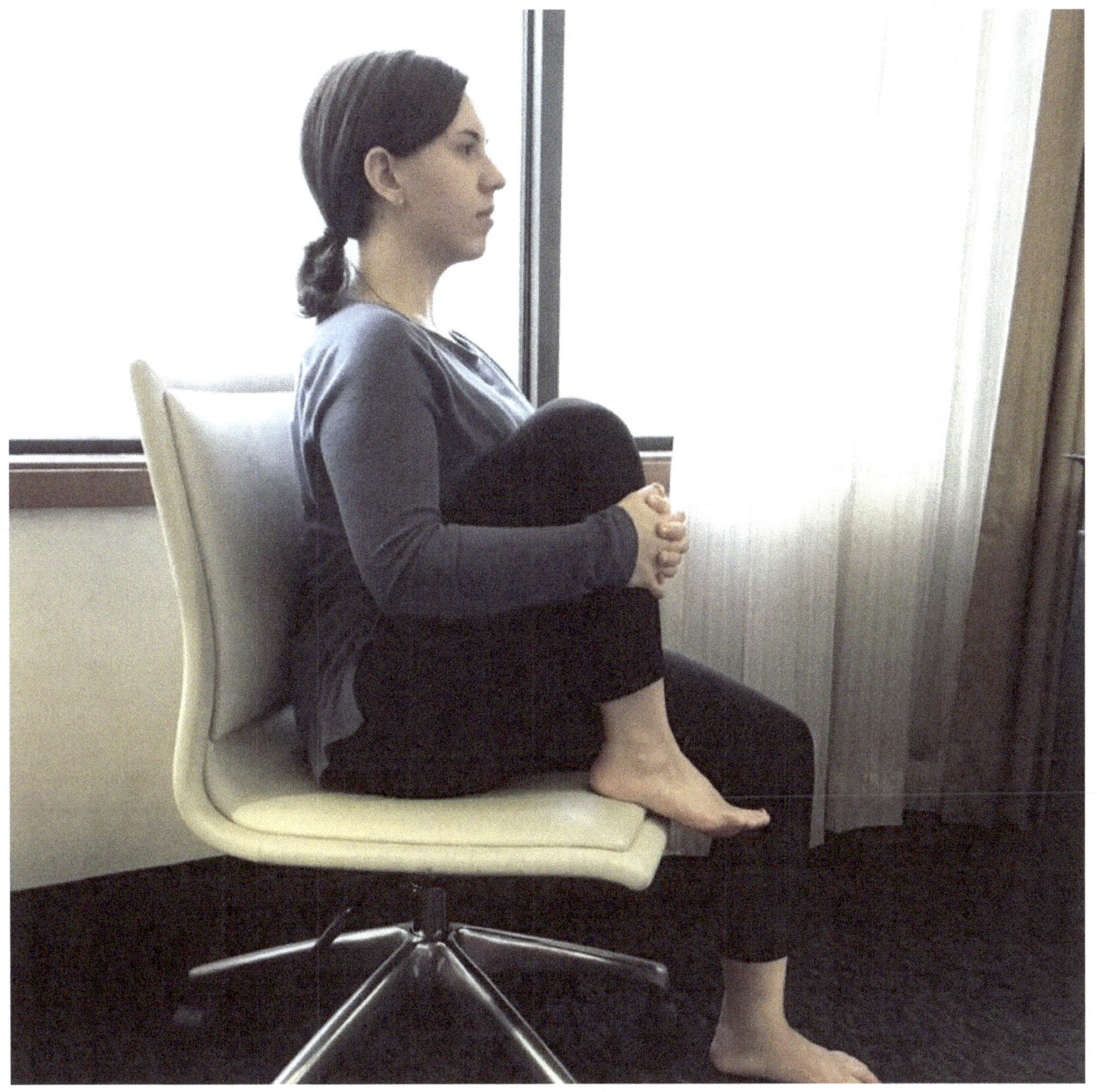

The Chair Knee to Chest Pose is a yoga posture that combines elements of balance, flexibility, and strength. It is a variation of the traditional Knee to Chest Pose, with the added support of a chair for balance and stability.

INSTRUCTION

1. Sit tall with feet flat on the floor.
2. Inhale, lift one knee towards your chest, hugging it with both arms.
3. Hold for a few breaths, then switch sides.

MISTAKES TO AVOID

1. Maintain an upright posture to avoid strain on the lower back.
2. Keep shoulders relaxed and away from the ears to prevent tension.
3. Remember to breathe deeply and steadily to enhance relaxation and flexibility.
4. Avoid excessive arching of the spine by engaging core muscles.
5. Perform the stretch slowly and smoothly to prevent injury.

Chair Butterfly Pose

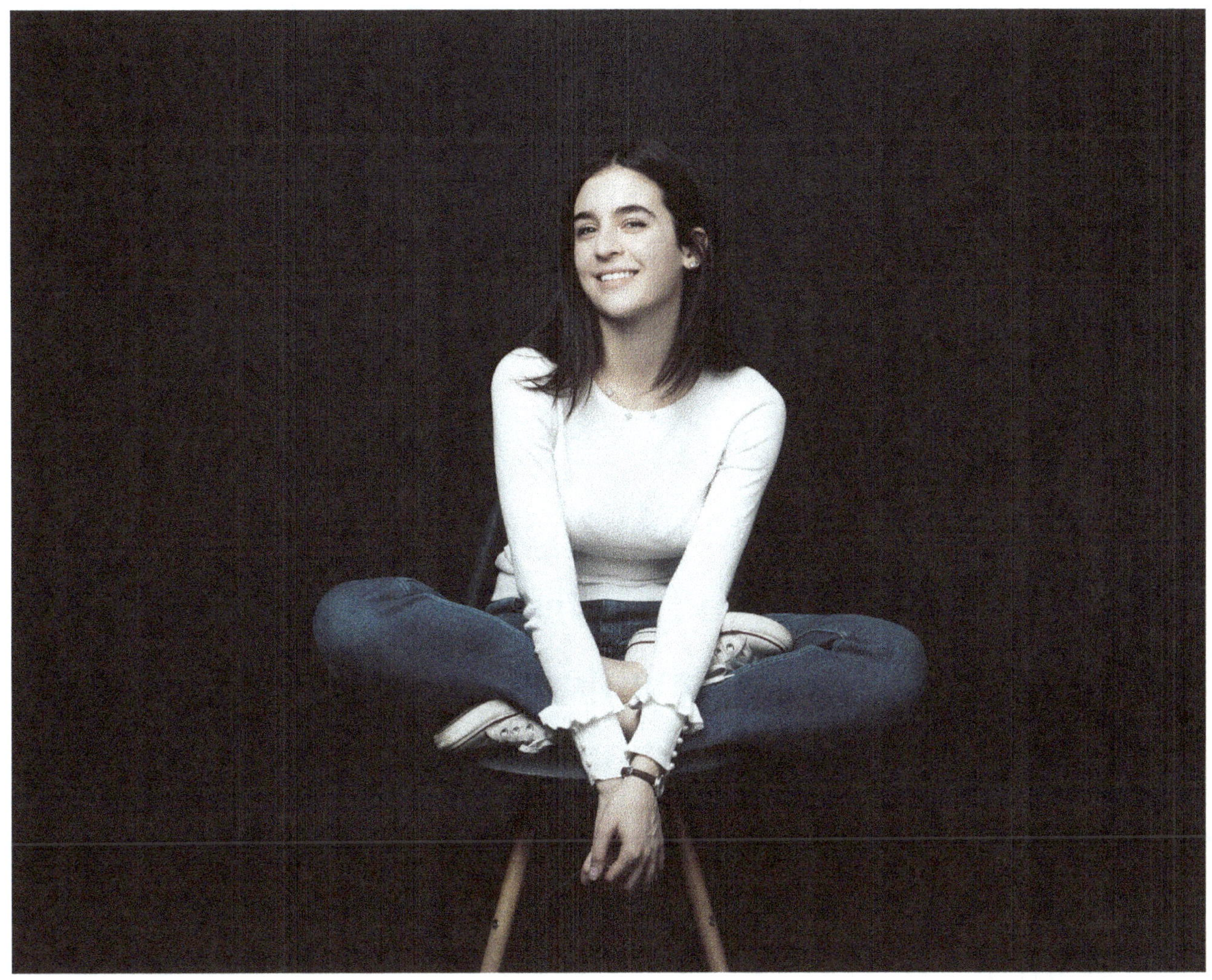

The Chair Butterfly Pose is a variation of the traditional Butterfly Pose, also known as Baddha Konasana in Sanskrit. In this variation, you sit on the edge of a chair instead of on the floor.

INSTRUCTION

1. Sit tall with feet flat on the floor, soles of the feet together.
2. Hold onto your feet or ankles with your hands.
3. Inhale, lengthen your spine.
4. Exhale, gently press your knees towards the floor, feeling a stretch in the inner thighs.

MISTAKES TO AVOID

1. Ensure your front knee aligns with your ankle to prevent strain. Aim for a right angle.
2. Keep your torso straight and shoulders relaxed to avoid slouching and maintain stability.
3. Avoid excessive arching of your lower back by engaging your core and keeping your tailbone slightly tucked.
4. Maintain a steady breath flow to stay relaxed and focused during the pose, inhaling and exhaling deeply.

Chair Pigeon Pose

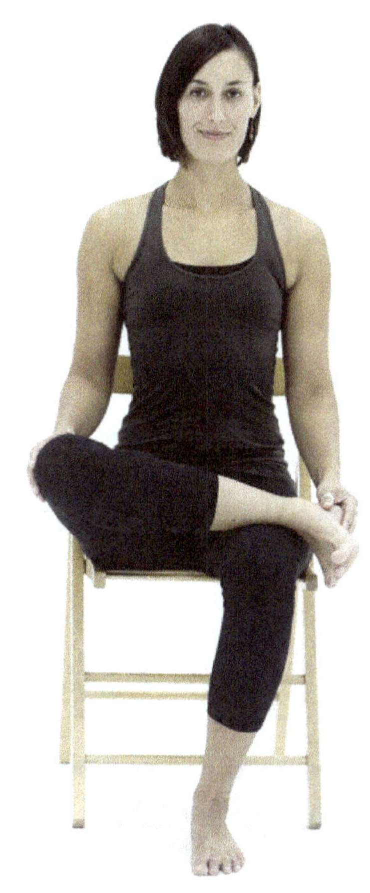

Chair Pigeon Pose is a variation of the traditional yoga pose called Pigeon Pose (Eka Pada Rajakapotasana). It combines elements of Chair Pose (Utkatasana) and Pigeon Pose to provide a deep stretch for the hips, groin, and thighs, while also engaging the muscles of the core and lower body for stability and balance.

INSTRUCTION

1. Sit tall with feet flat on the floor.
2. Cross your right ankle over your left thigh, flexing your right foot.
3. Keep your spine long and hinge forward slightly, feeling a stretch in the outer hip.
4. Hold for a few breaths, then switch sides.

MISTAKES TO AVOID

1. Ensure your bent leg is parallel to the front of the chair to avoid strain.
2. Maintain an upright posture to prevent pressure on the lower back.
3. Avoid forcing your bent knee too far sideways to prevent discomfort.
4. Remember to breathe deeply and steadily to enhance relaxation and flexibility.
5. Use the chair for support if needed to maintain stability throughout the pose.

Chair Hamstring Stretch

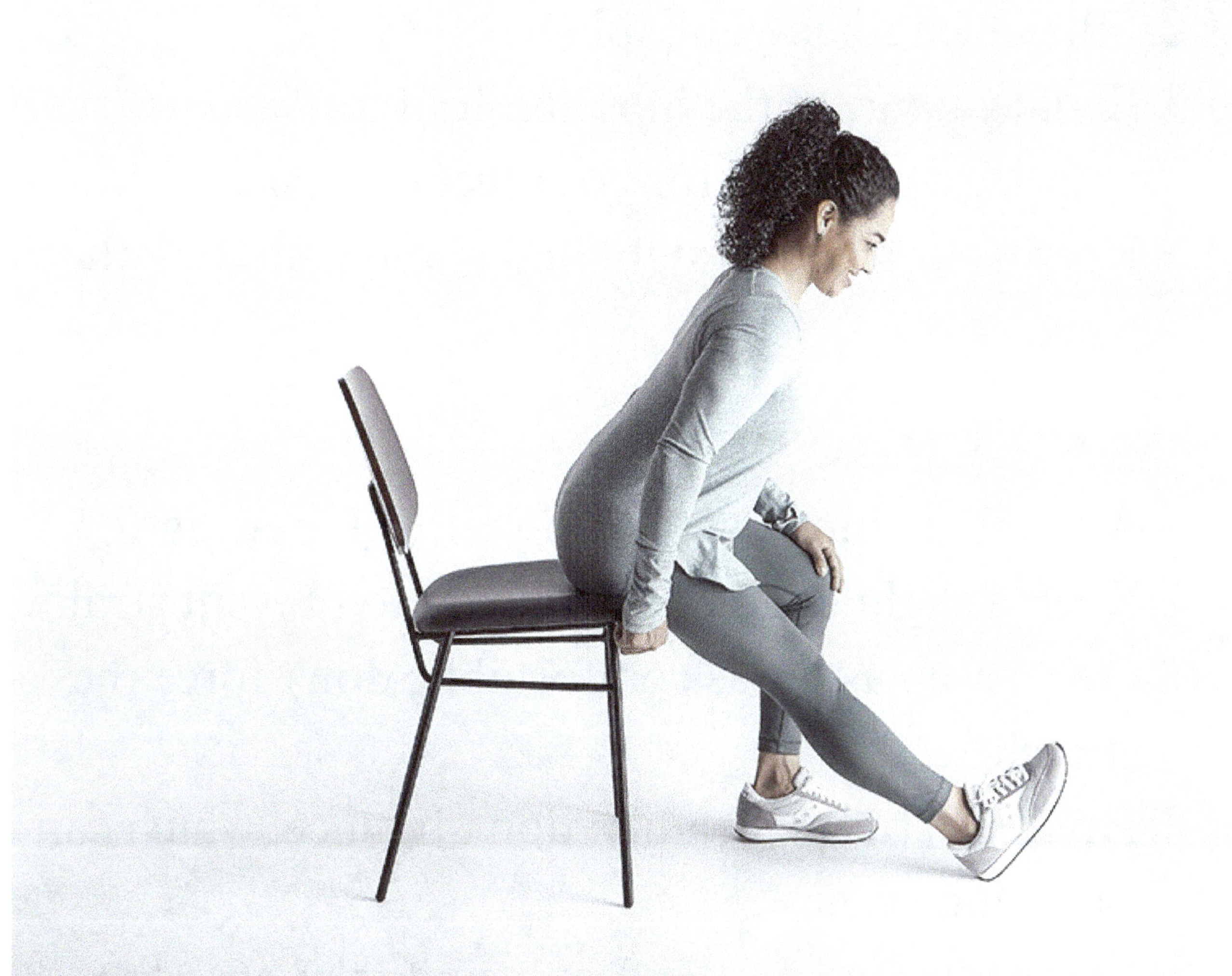

The Chair Hamstring Stretch is a stretching exercise that specifically targets the hamstring muscles, which are located on the back of your thighs. This stretch can be performed while sitting on a chair, making it a convenient option for individuals who may have difficulty with traditional standing or floor-based hamstring stretches.

INSTRUCTION

1. Sit tall with legs extended.
2. Inhale, lengthen your spine.
3. Exhale, hinge at the hips and fold forward over your legs, reaching for your feet or shins.
4. Keep your spine straight and avoid rounding the back.

MISTAKES TO AVOID

1. Avoid hunching over; keep your spine straight.
2. Keep a slight bend in your knees to prevent strain.
3. Only reach as far as comfortable; don't force the stretch.
4. Hold the stretch steadily; don't bounce, which can cause injury.
5. Remember to breathe deeply and relax into the stretch.

Chair Leg Extension

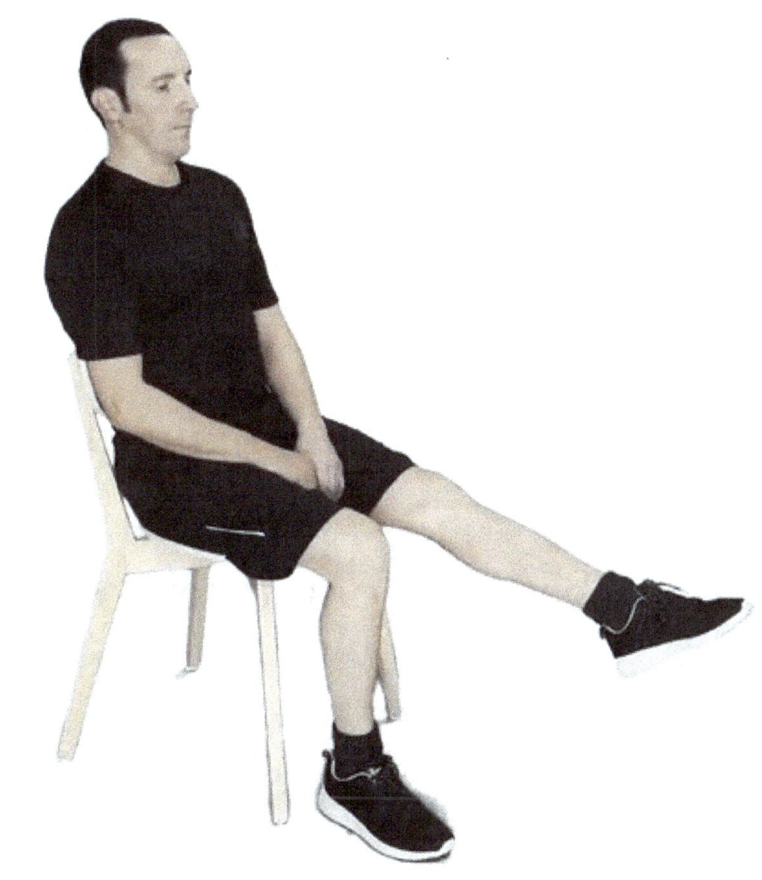

The seated leg extension is a strength training exercise primarily targeting the quadriceps muscles of the thighs.

INSTRUCTION

1. Sit tall with legs extended.
2. Flex your feet, engage your quadriceps, and point your toes towards your body.
3. Hold for a few breaths, feeling a stretch in the calves and hamstrings.

MISTAKES TO AVOID

1. Avoid hunching forward to maintain proper posture.
2. Keep a slight bend in your knees to prevent strain on the joints.
3. Avoid pushing your leg too far out, stay within a comfortable range.
4. Remember to breathe steadily throughout the exercise.
5. Ensure your leg is extended in line with your hip to maximize effectiveness.

Chair Forward Fold with Twist

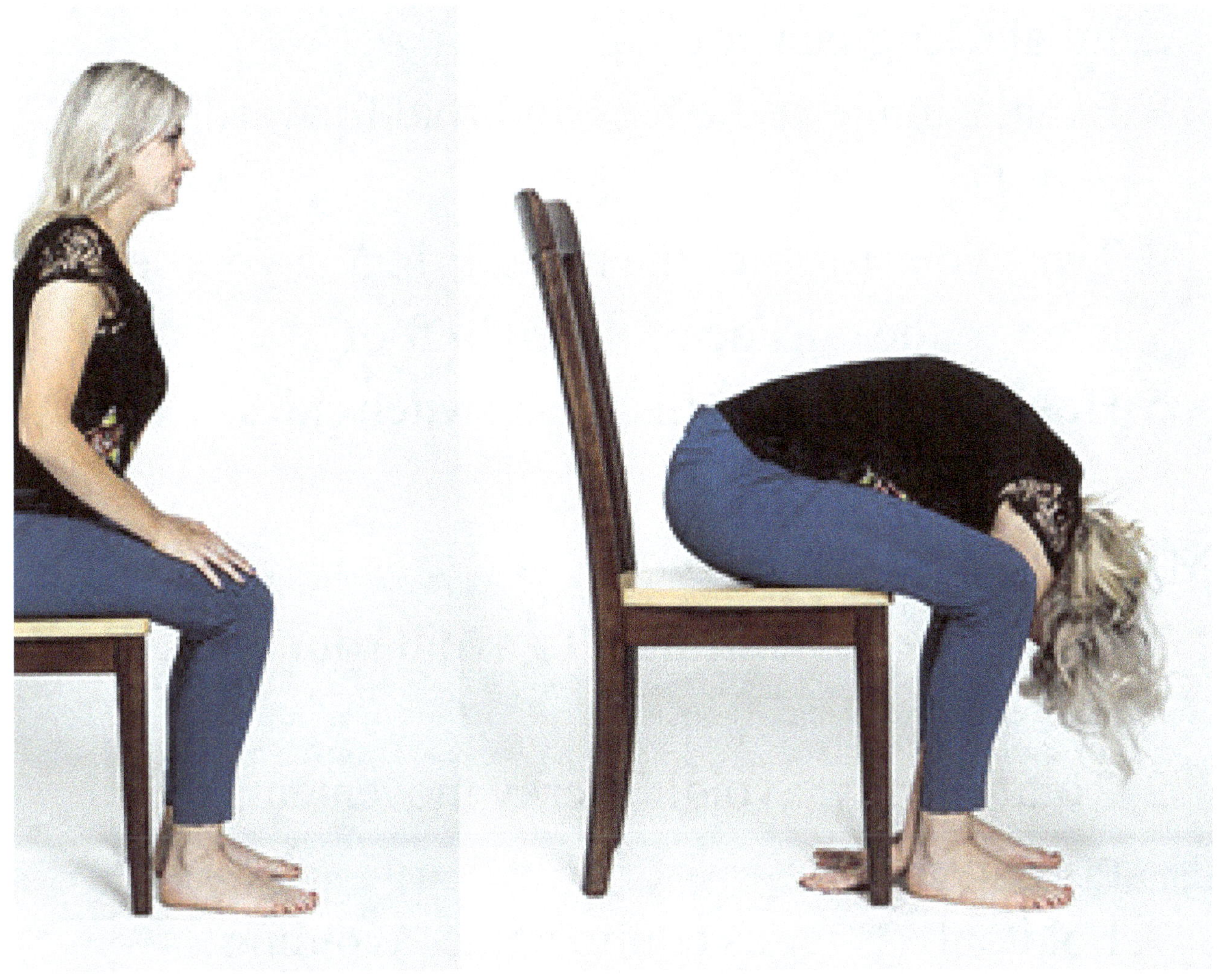

The seated forward fold with twist is a yoga pose that combines elements of forward bending and spinal rotation.

INSTRUCTION

1. Sit tall with legs extended.
2. Inhale, lengthen your spine.
3. Exhale, hinge at the hips and fold forward over your legs.
4. Twist your torso to the right, bringing your left hand to the outside of the right foot.
5. Hold for a few breaths, then switch sides.

MISTAKES TO AVOID

1. Keep your spine straight to avoid rounding excessively.
2. Rotate gently, avoiding jerky movements to prevent strain.
3. Fold only as far as comfortable, avoiding overstretching.
4. Keep a slight bend to protect your knee joints.
5. Remember to breathe deeply throughout the stretch for relaxation.

Chair Cow Face Pose

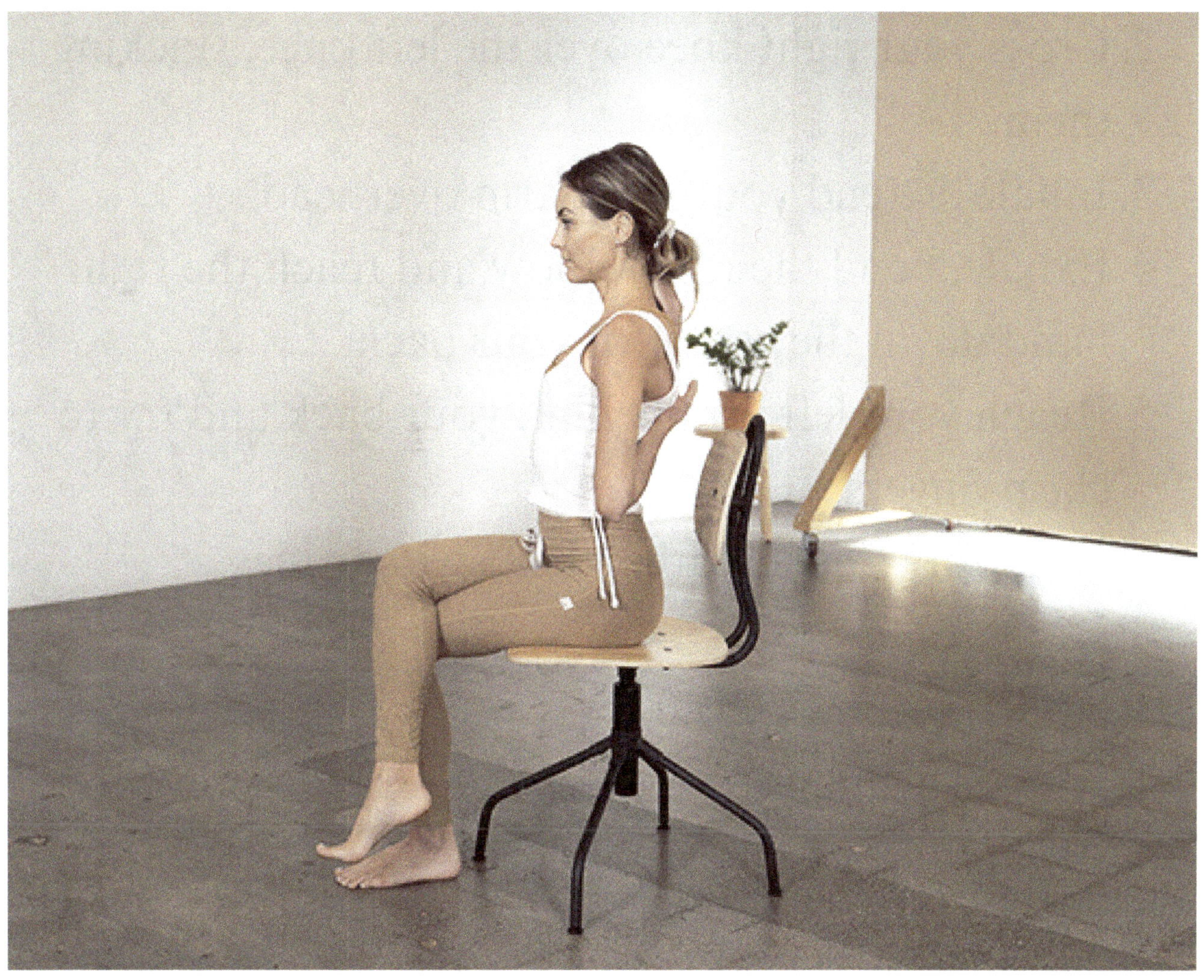

The Seated Cow Face Pose, known as Gomukhasana in Sanskrit, is a yoga asana (pose) that stretches and opens up various parts of the body, particularly the hips, thighs, shoulders, and chest.

INSTRUCTION

1. Sit tall with knees bent and feet flat on the floor.
2. Cross your right knee over the left knee, stacking them.
3. Inhale, extend your right arm overhead.
4. Exhale, bend the right elbow and reach the right hand down the center of your back.
5. Reach your left arm behind your back and try to clasp fingers.
6. Hold for a few breaths, then switch sides.

MISTAKES TO AVOID

1. Avoid stacking your knees unevenly to prevent strain.
2. Keep your spine tall and avoid slouching forward to protect your posture.
3. Don't force your hands to touch if they don't naturally reach; use a strap if needed.
4. Relax your shoulders away from your ears to release tension.
5. Remember to breathe deeply and evenly throughout the pose for relaxation.

Chair Garland Pose

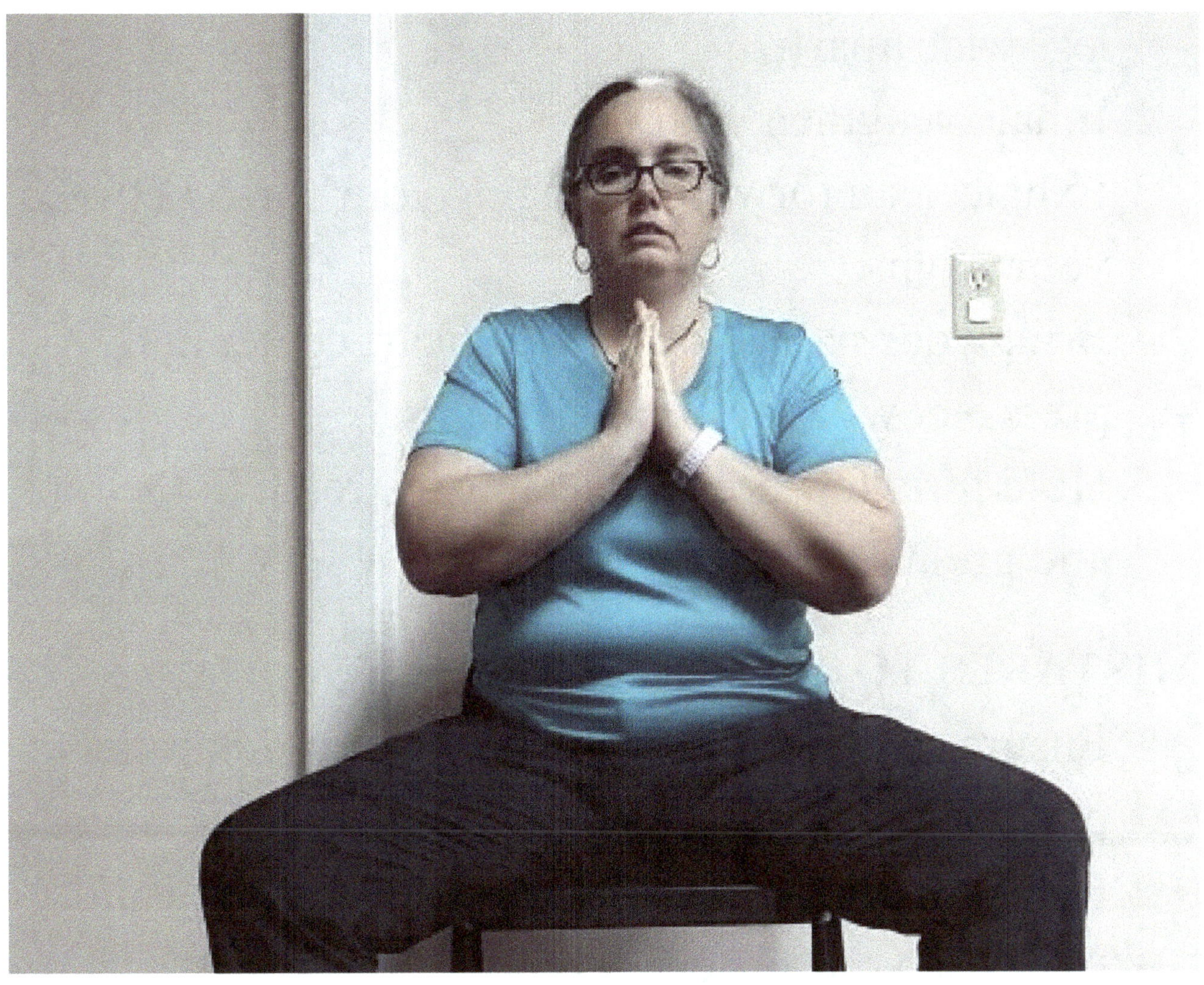

The seated Garland Pose, also known as Malasana in Sanskrit, is a yoga pose that involves squatting while seated. Seated Garland Pose is great for stretching the hips, groin, and lower back, and it can also help improve flexibility and mobility in these areas.

INSTRUCTION

1. Sit tall with feet flat on the floor, knees bent, and legs wide apart.
2. Inhale, lengthen your spine.
3. Exhale, lean forward, bringing your torso between your thighs.
4. Bring your palms together at heart center and press elbows against inner thighs.
5. Hold for a few breaths, feeling a stretch in the hips and groin.

MISTAKES TO AVOID

1. Ensure your feet are firmly planted and parallel to prevent instability.
2. Keep your spine straight to avoid slouching and strain on your lower back.
3. Lift your chest to open up the front body and avoid compressing the chest and lungs.
4. Relax your shoulders away from your ears to release tension and improve posture.

Chair Reclined Twist

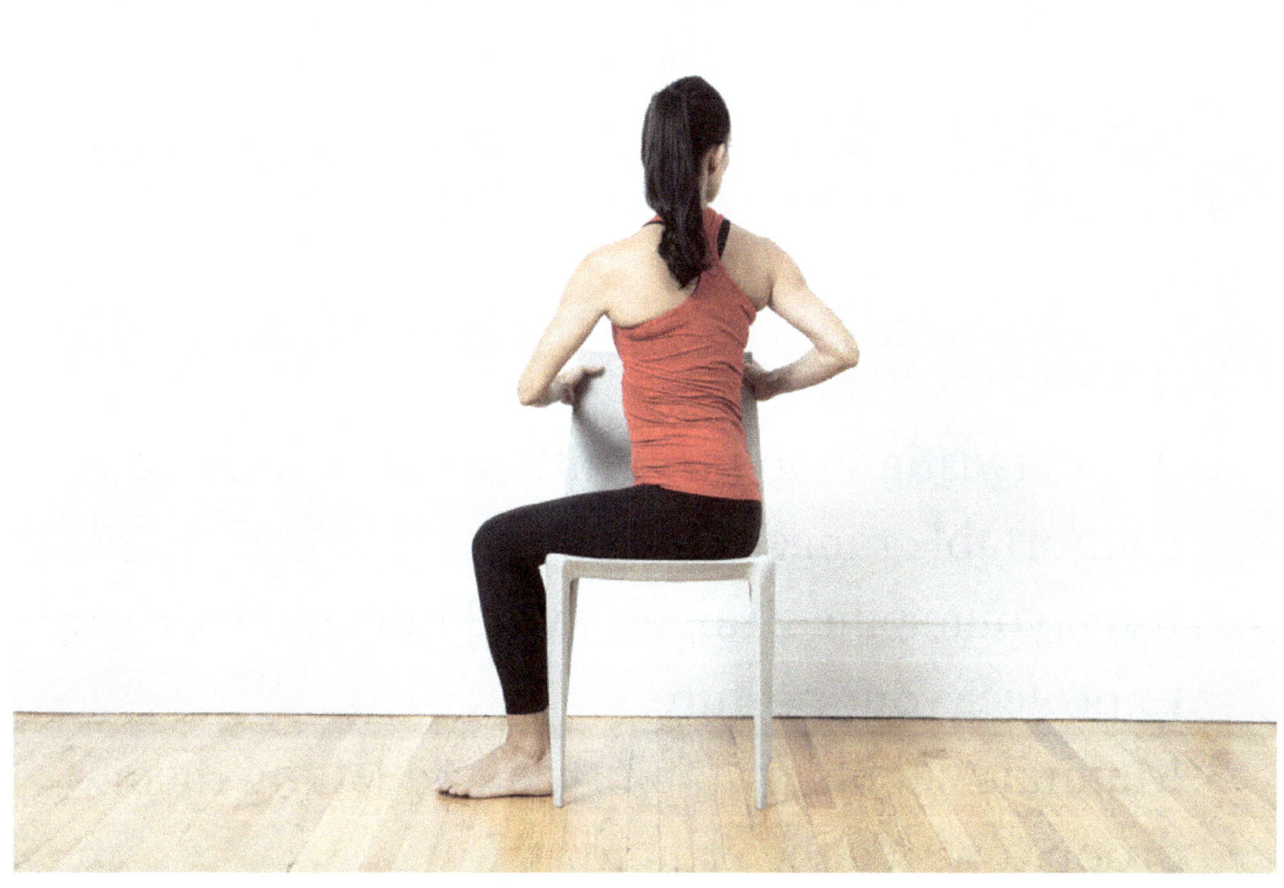

Chair Reclined Twist" is likely a yoga pose or exercise that combines elements of seated or reclined postures with a twisting motion.

INSTRUCTION

1. Sit tall with legs extended.
2. Inhale, lengthen your spine.
3. Exhale, twist your torso to the right, bringing your left hand to the outside of the right knee and your right hand behind you.
4. Hold for a few breaths, then switch sides.

MISTAKES TO AVOID

1. Avoid twisting too far; gently rotate within your comfortable range.
2. Keep your spine straight; avoid hunching forward to protect your posture.
3. Maintain shoulder stability; avoid letting them droop towards the ground.
4. Remember to breathe deeply; inhale to lengthen the spine and exhale to deepen the twist.
5. Keep your neck aligned with your spine; avoid craning it too far in the twist.

Chair Side Plank

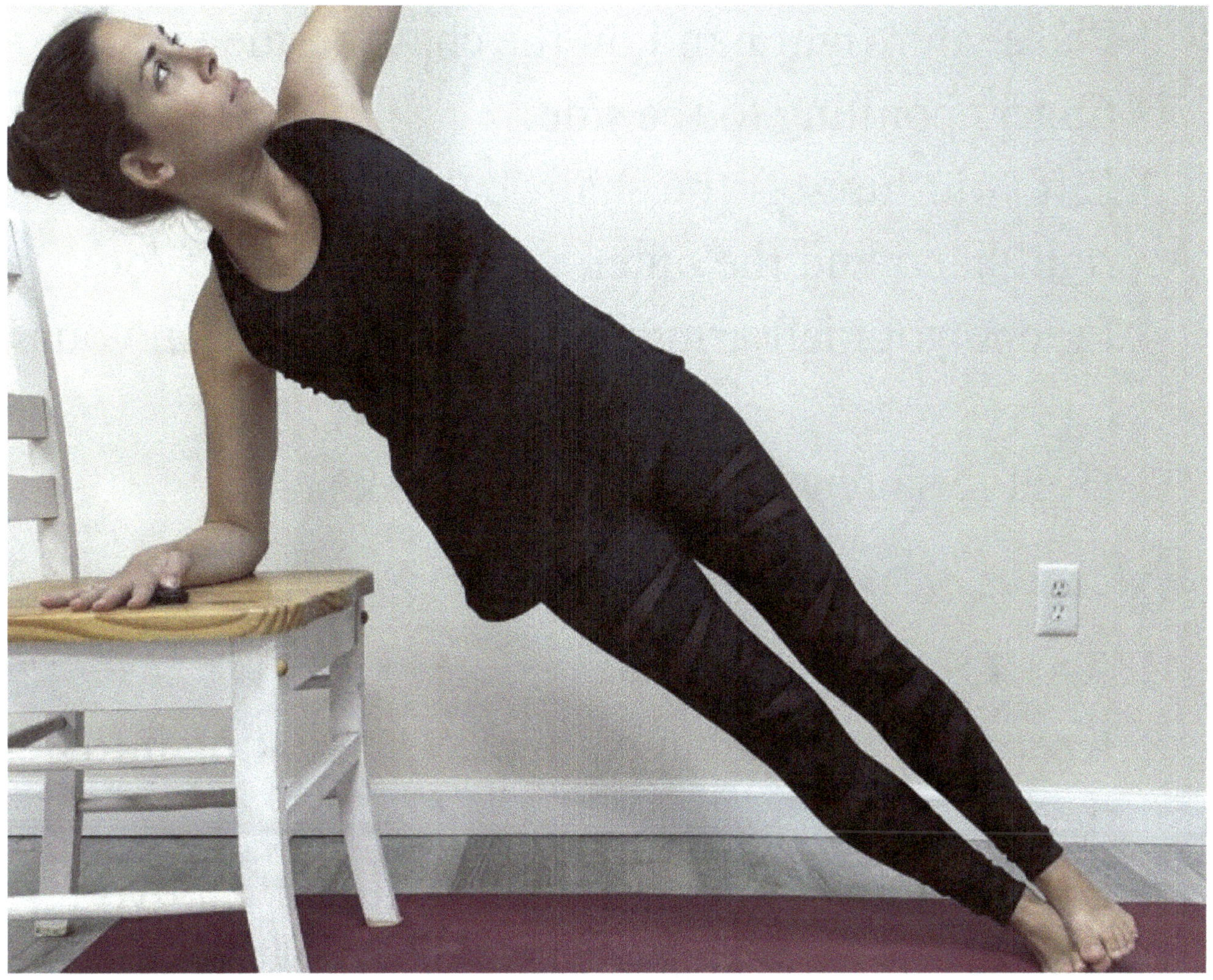

The Chair Side Plank is a variation of the traditional side plank exercise, which is commonly performed to strengthen the muscles of the core, particularly the obliques, as well as the shoulders, hips, and legs. The chair adds an extra element of instability and challenge to the exercise.

INSTRUCTION

1. Sit tall with legs extended.
2. Place your right hand on the chair beside you, fingers pointing to the side.
3. Lift your hips off the chair, balancing on your right hand and the outer edge of your right foot.
4. Extend your left arm overhead or place it on your hip.
5. Hold for a few breaths, then switch sides.

MISTAKES TO AVOID

1. Keep your core engaged to prevent sinking into the hips.
2. Ensure your shoulder is stacked directly above your wrist to avoid strain.
3. Maintain a straight line from head to heels to prevent sinking or lifting the hips.
4. Distribute weight evenly between your hand and feet to avoid tipping over.
5. Remember to breathe steadily to maintain relaxation and focus.

Chair Downward Facing Dog

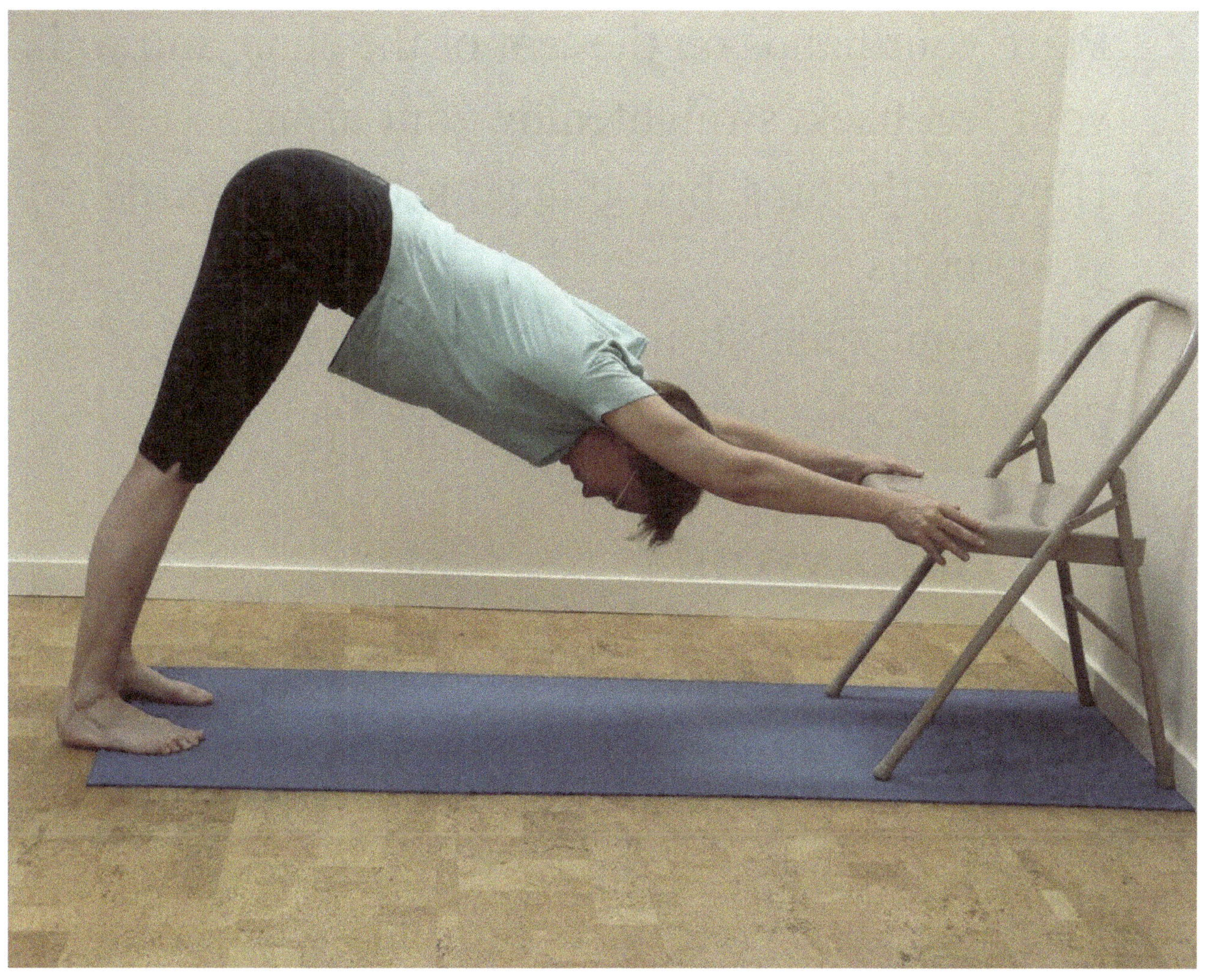

Chair Downward Facing Dog" is a yoga pose that combines elements of both Chair Pose (Utkatasana) and Downward Facing Dog Pose (Adho Mukha Svanasana). It's a variation that offers a unique combination of strength, flexibility, and balance.

INSTRUCTION

1. Sit tall with feet flat on the floor.
2. Place your hands on the seat of the chair and walk your feet back, straightening your arms.
3. Hinge at the hips, bringing your torso towards your thighs.
4. Keep your spine straight and legs engaged, pressing heels towards the floor.

MISTAKES TO AVOID

1. Keep your spine straight, avoiding rounding to prevent strain.
2. Relax your shoulders away from your ears to avoid tension.
3. Maintain an open chest to prevent compressing your lungs.
4. Keep a slight bend in your knees to avoid hyperextension.
5. Ensure your hands are firmly planted and feet hip-width apart for balance.

Chair Cobra Pose

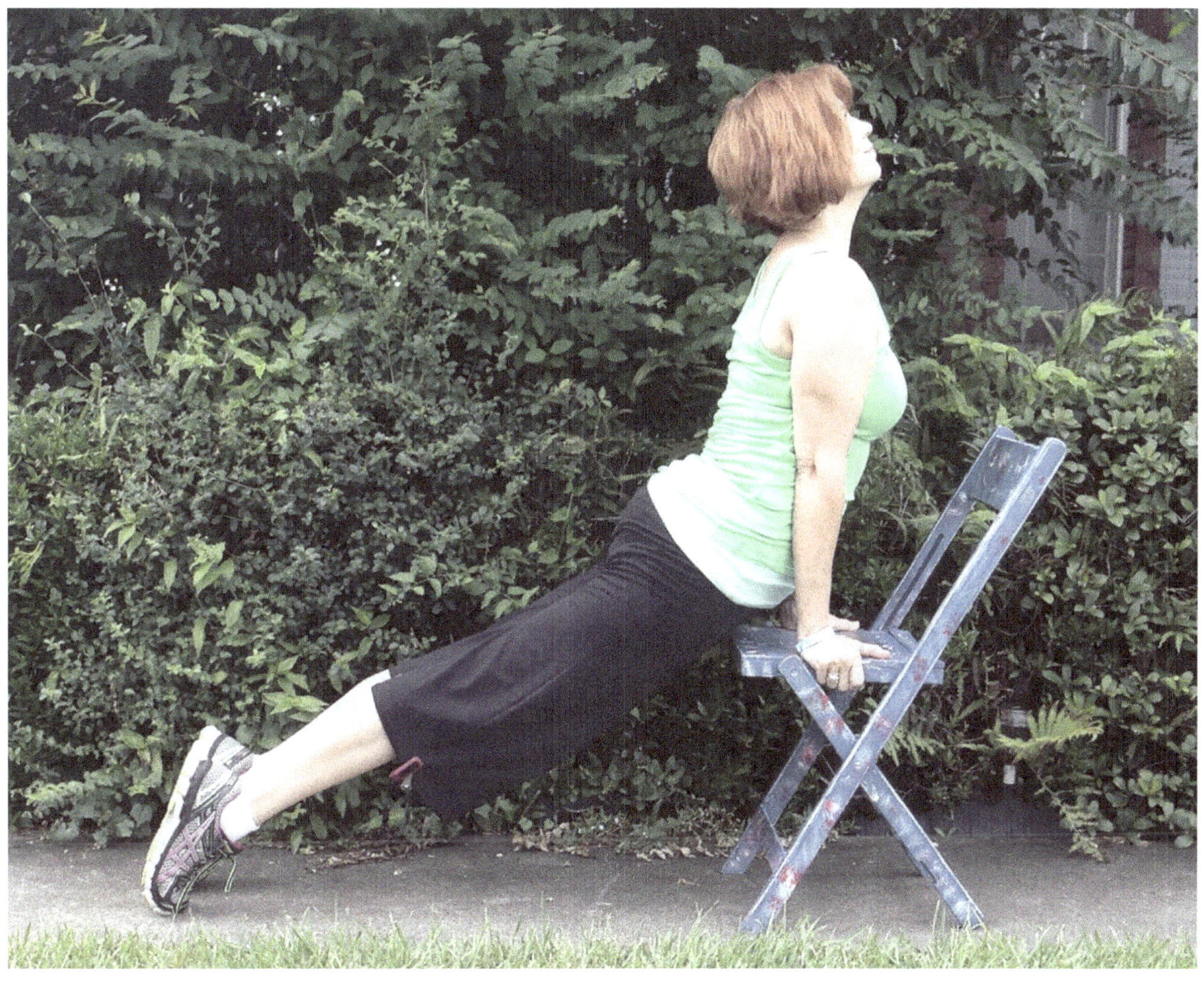

The Chair Cobra Pose is a yoga posture that combines elements of both the Utkatasana (Chair Pose) and the Bhujangasana (Cobra Pose). It's a variation that challenges balance, strength, and flexibility while providing benefits for the back, spine, and core muscles.

INSTRUCTION

1. Sit tall with feet flat on the floor.
2. Place your hands on the seat of the chair, shoulder-width apart.
3. Inhale, press into your hands, and lift your chest, arching your back slightly.
4. Keep shoulders relaxed away from ears and gaze forward.

MISTAKES TO AVOID

1. Avoid craning your neck upwards too far.
2. Keep shoulders away from ears to prevent tension.
3. Avoid excessive arching of the spine.
4. Keep a slight bend in the elbows to prevent strain.
5. Remember to breathe steadily throughout the pose.

Chair Upward Facing Dog

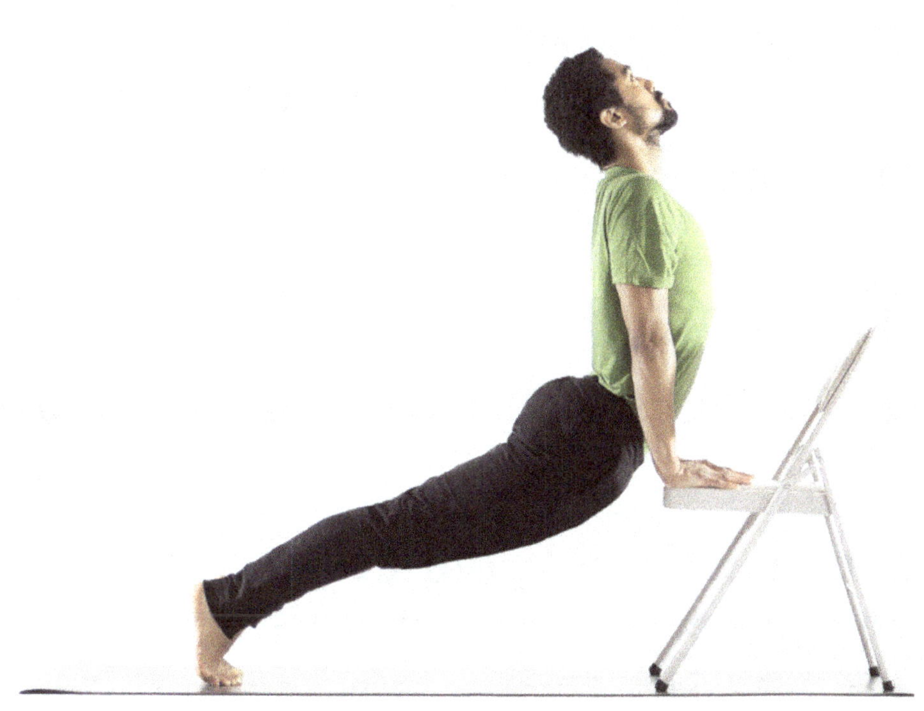

hair Upward Facing Dog" is likely a combination or variation of yoga poses, specifically blending aspects of "Chair Pose" (Utkatasana) and "Upward Facing Dog" (Urdhva Mukha Svanasana).

INSTRUCTION

1. Sit tall with feet flat on the floor.
2. Place your hands on the seat of the chair behind you, fingers pointing towards your body.
3. Inhale, press into your hands, and lift your chest, opening through the front of the body.
4. Keep shoulders relaxed away from ears and engage your core.

MISTAKES TO AVOID

1. Keep your shoulders away from your ears to avoid hunching.
2. Lift your chest and open your heart to avoid rounding your back.
3. Engage your core to prevent your hips from dropping too low.
4. Avoid hyperextending your lower back by keeping a slight tuck in your tailbone.

Chair Bridge Pose

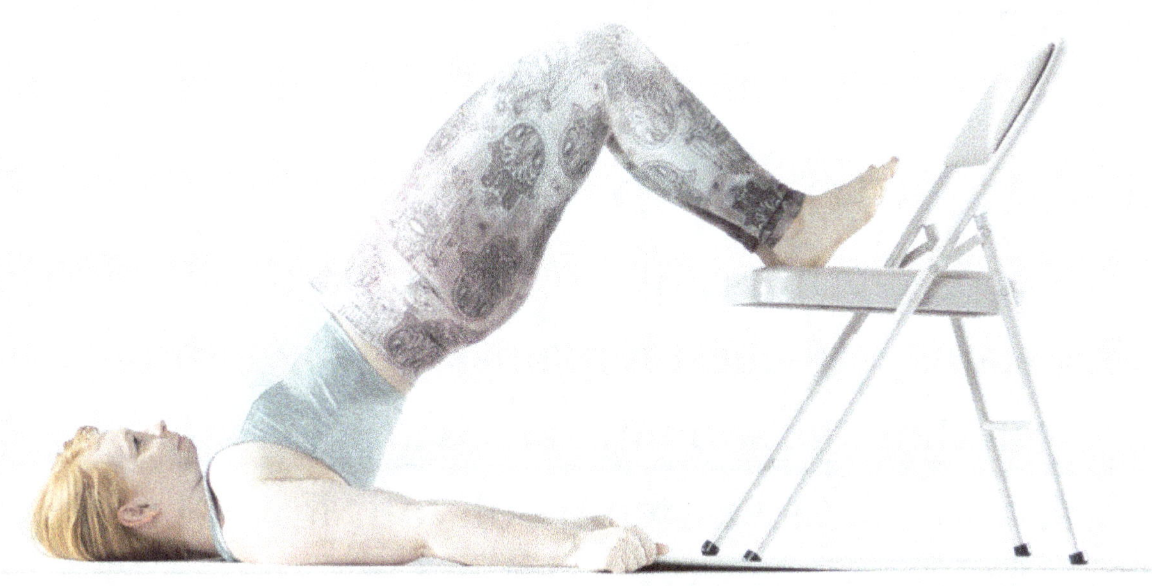

Chair Bridge Pose is a variation of the traditional Bridge Pose (Setu Bandhasana) in yoga. It combines the elements of both Chair Pose (Utkatasana) and Bridge Pose to create a unique posture that offers various benefits for the body.

INSTRUCTION

1. Sit tall with feet flat on the floor, hip-width apart.
2. Place your hands on the seat of the chair beside you, fingers pointing towards your body.
3. Inhale, press into your hands and feet, lifting your hips towards the ceiling.
4. Keep your spine long and engage your glutes and hamstrings.

MISTAKES TO AVOID

1. Keep your hips lifted to maintain the bridge shape.
2. Ensure your chest remains open, avoiding rounding the shoulders forward.
3. Avoid excessive arching of your lower back by engaging your core.
4. Ensure your feet are hip-width apart and firmly planted on the ground.
5. Remember to breathe continuously and deeply throughout the pose.

Chair Camel Pose

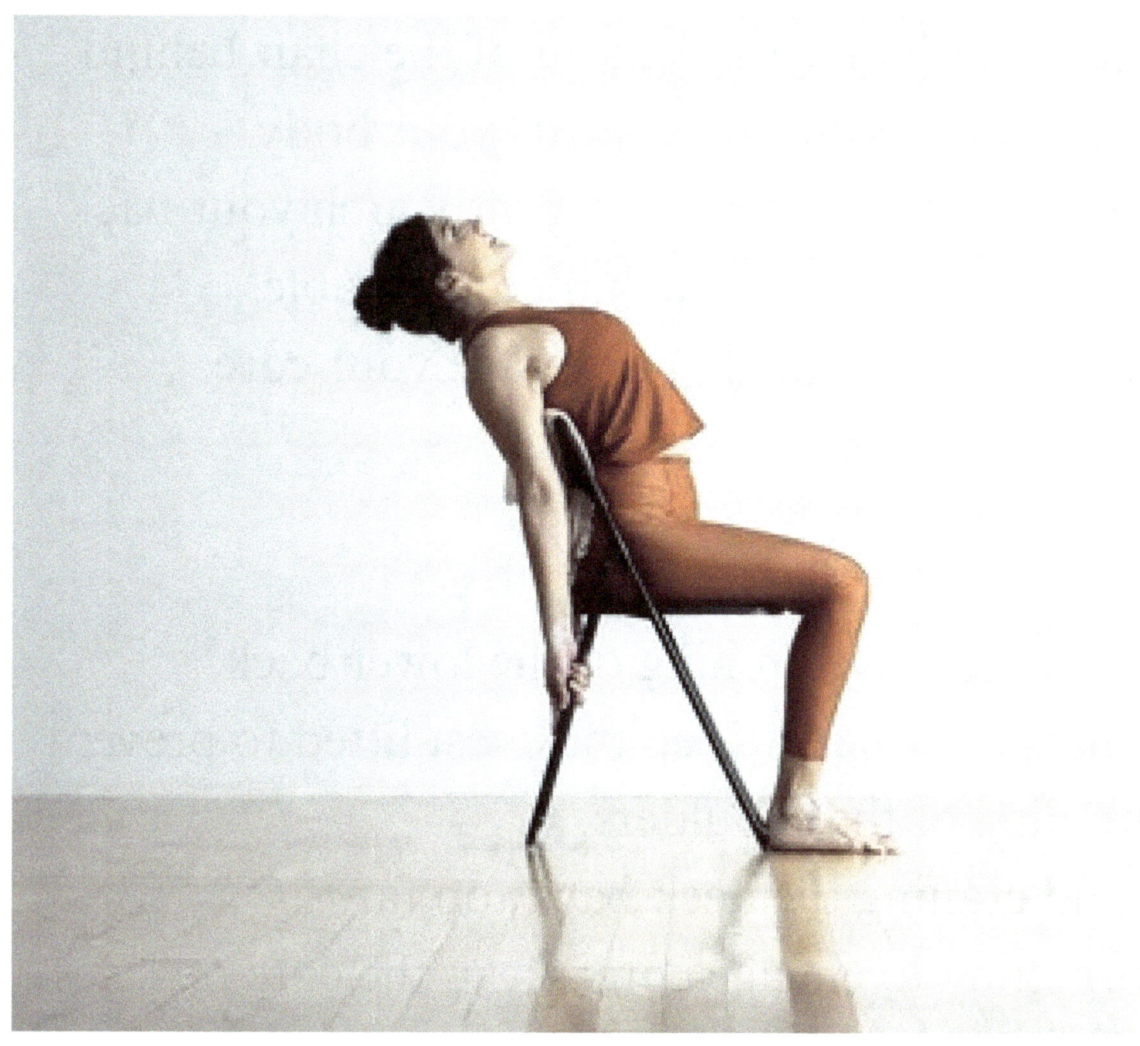

Chair Camel Pose is a variation of the traditional Camel Pose (Ustrasana) in yoga. It combines the benefits of Ustrasana with the stability and support provided by a chair.

INSTRUCTION

1. Sit tall with knees bent and feet flat on the floor.
2. Place your hands on the seat of the chair behind you, fingers pointing towards your body.
3. Inhale, lift your chest, and gently arch your back, dropping your head back if comfortable.
4. Keep hips grounded and engage your core.

MISTAKES TO AVOID

1. Avoid excessive arching of the lower back.
2. Collapsing Chest: Keep the chest lifted to prevent rounding of the shoulders.
3. Avoid craning the neck back too far.
4. Forgetting to engage core: Keep the core muscles engaged to support the back.

Chair Locust Pose

Chair Locust Pose" is not a commonly recognized yoga pose in traditional yoga practices. It seems like it might be a hybrid or a variation of two different poses: "Chair Pose" (Utkatasana) and "Locust Pose" (Salabhasana).

INSTRUCTION

1. Sit tall with feet flat on the floor.
2. Place your hands on the seat of the chair beside you, fingers pointing towards your body.
3. Inhale, lift your chest, and extend your legs straight back, lifting them off the floor.
4. Keep your gaze forward and engage your glutes and hamstrings.

MISTAKES TO AVOID

1. Avoid letting your lower back arch excessively.
2. Keep your gaze forward to prevent tension in the neck.
3. Lift only as far as comfortable to prevent straining your back.
4. Remember to breathe steadily throughout the pose.
5. Keep your shoulders relaxed and away from your ears.

Chair Bow Pose

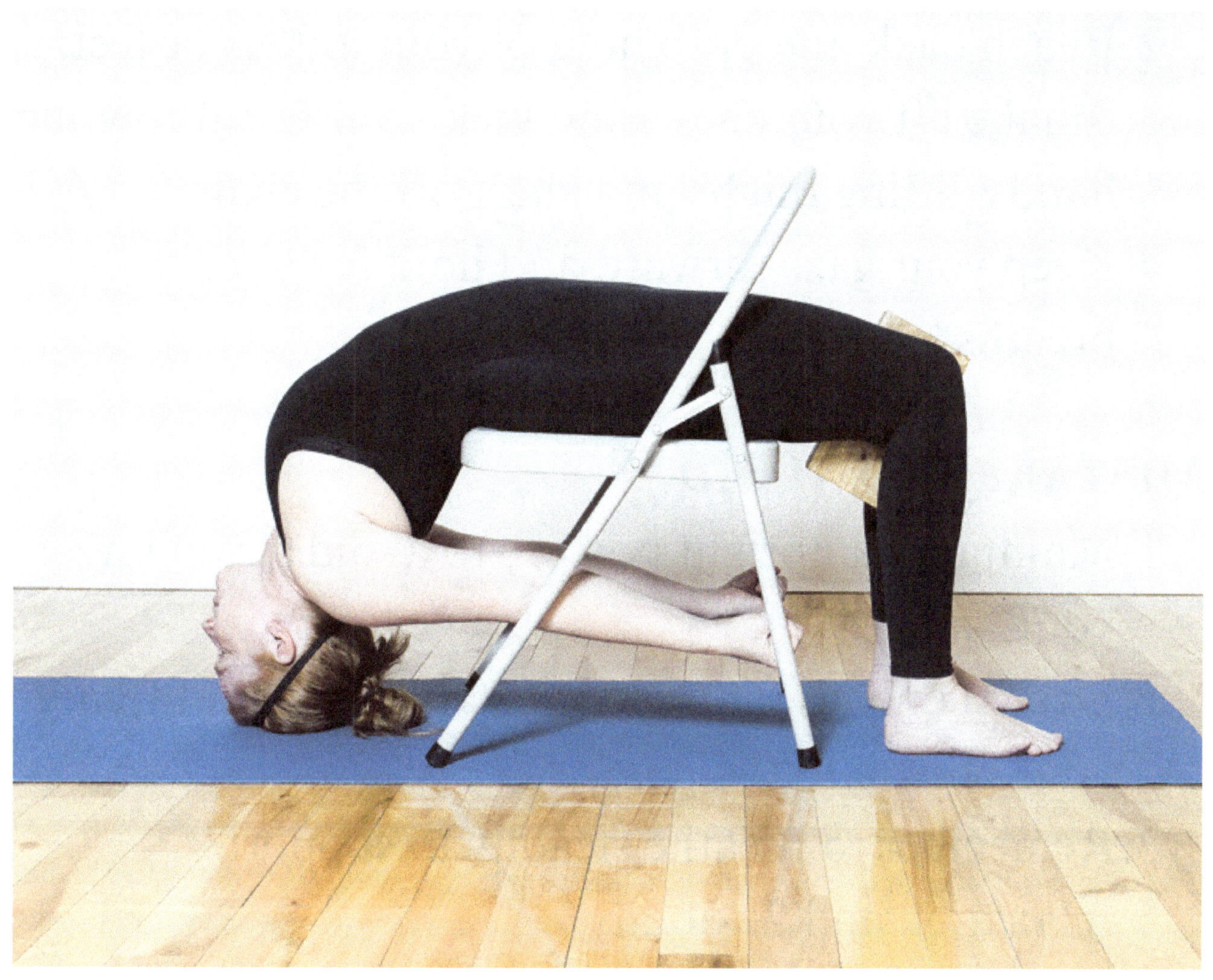

Chair Bow Pose, also known as Utkatasana Dhanurasana, is a yoga pose that combines elements of both Chair Pose (Utkatasana) and Bow Pose (Dhanurasana). It's a challenging and advanced variation that requires flexibility, strength, and balance.

INSTRUCTION

1. Sit tall with knees bent and feet flat on the floor.
2. Reach back and grab hold of your ankles or feet.
3. Inhale, lift your chest, and kick your feet into your hands, lifting thighs and chest off the chair.
4. Keep your gaze forward and hold for a few breaths.

MISTAKES TO AVOID

1. Maintain an upright posture to avoid strain on your back.
2. Stretch only as far as comfortable without forcing your body into the pose.
3. Remember to breathe steadily to support relaxation and flexibility.
4. Avoid tensing your hands on the chair; instead, focus on grounding through your feet.
5. Keep shoulders relaxed to prevent tension in the neck and upper back.

Chair Half Moon Pose

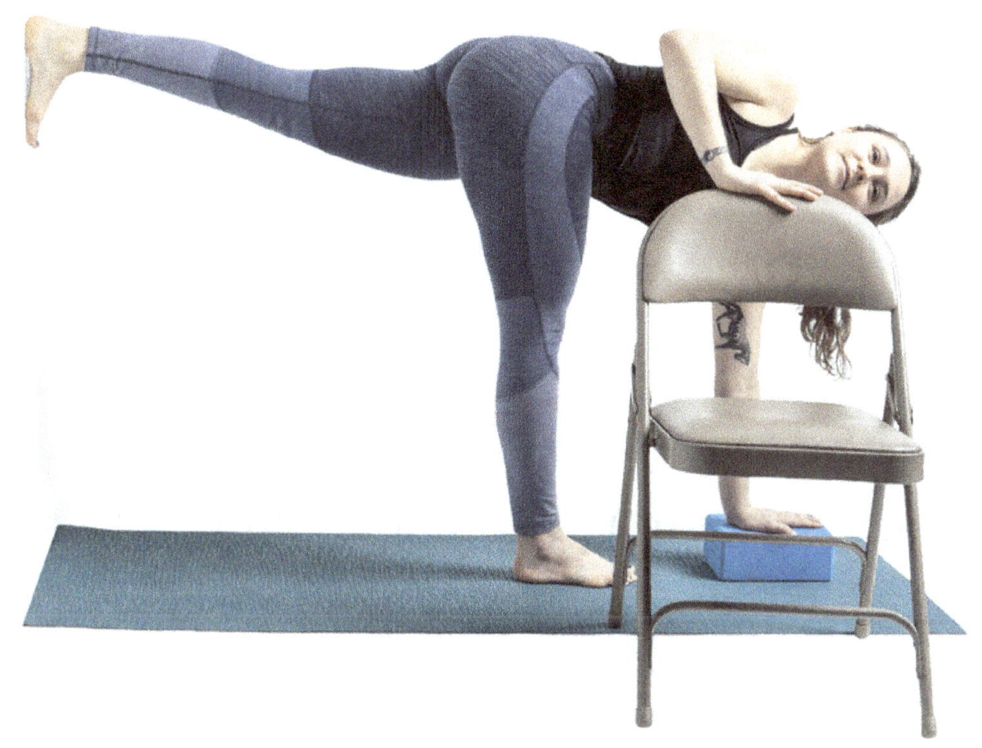

Chair Half Moon Pose, also known as Ardha Chandrasana in Sanskrit, is a variation of the traditional Half Moon Pose (Ardha Chandrasana). It combines elements of balance, strength, and flexibility, making it a challenging yet rewarding yoga posture.

INSTRUCTION

1. Sit tall with feet flat on the floor.
2. Extend your right leg out to the side, keeping foot flexed.
3. Lean to the right, placing your right hand on the chair seat.
4. Extend your left arm overhead, creating a half moon shape with your body.
5. Hold for a few breaths, then switch sides.

MISTAKES TO AVOID

1. Focus on grounding your standing foot and engaging your core for stability.
2. Keep your chest open and spine straight to prevent rounding and strain in your back.
3. Ensure your hips remain stacked and avoid tilting to the side to maintain proper alignment.
4. Avoid excessive arching or rounding of your spine by maintaining a neutral position.
5. Extend your arm overhead in line with your body to avoid strain on your shoulder and maintain balance.

Chair Revolved Triangle Pose

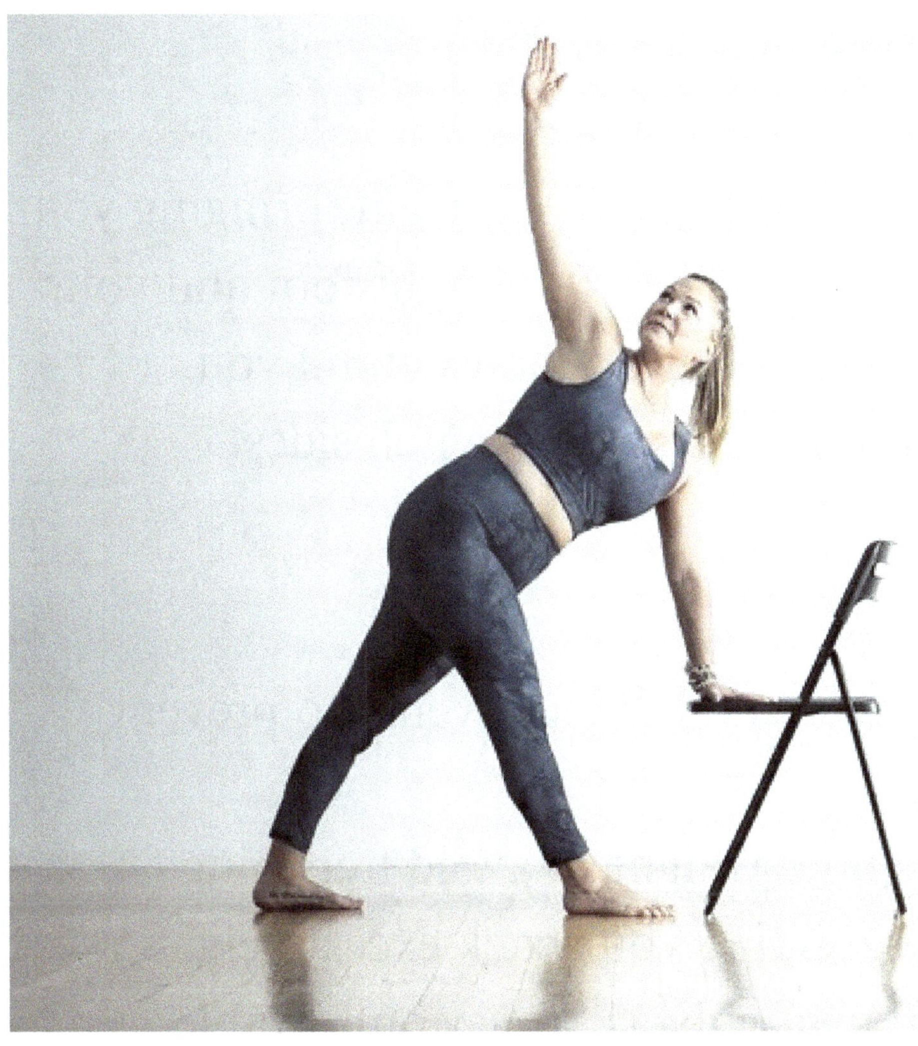

The Chair Revolved Triangle Pose, also known as Parivrtta Utkatasana in Sanskrit, is a variation of the Chair Pose (Utkatasana) combined with the Revolved Triangle Pose (Parivrtta Trikonasana). It's a challenging yoga posture that requires balance, strength, and flexibility.

INSTRUCTION

1. Sit tall with legs extended.
2. Open your legs wide apart.
3. Inhale, lengthen your spine.
4. Exhale, twist your torso to the right, bringing your left hand to the outside of the right foot and your right hand to the floor or chair behind you.
5. Hold for a few breaths, then switch sides.

MISTAKES TO AVOID

1. Secure your feet and balance evenly to prevent wobbling.
2. Keep your spine straight to avoid hunching forward or rounding your back excessively.
3. Extend your arm only as far as comfortable without straining to maintain balance and prevent overstretching.
4. Ensure both hips face forward to avoid twisting excessively, which could strain your lower back.

Chair Revolved Lunge

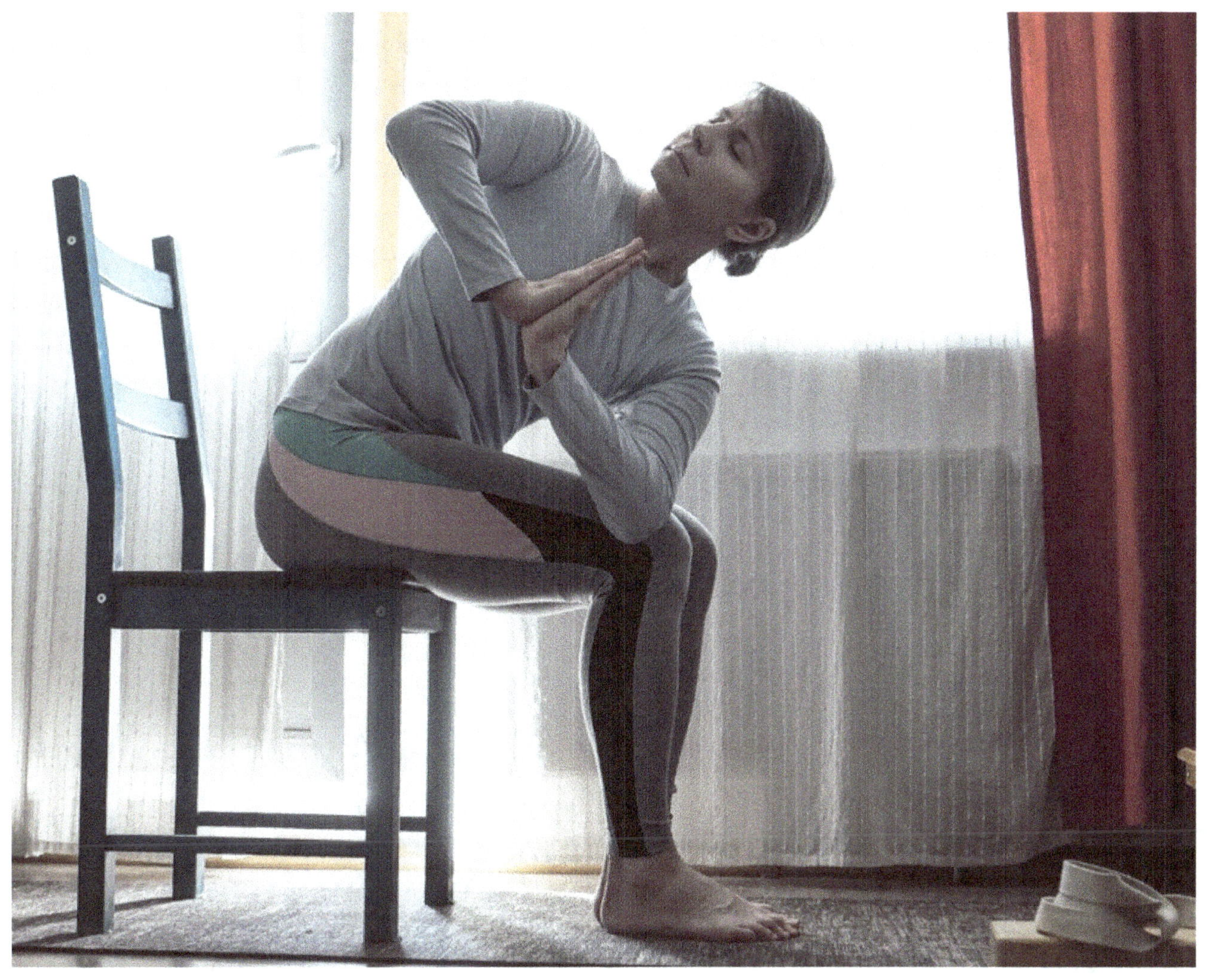

The Chair Revolved Lunge is a yoga pose that combines elements of balance, strength, and flexibility. It is a variation of the traditional Revolved Lunge pose, with the addition of a chair for support and stability.

INSTRUCTION

1. Sit tall with feet flat on the floor.
2. Extend your right leg back, keeping toes tucked under.
3. Inhale, raise your arms overhead.
4. Exhale, twist your torso to the right, bringing your left hand to the outside of the right knee and your right hand behind you.
5. Hold for a few breaths, then switch sides.

MISTAKES TO AVOID

1. Avoid over-rotating your torso, keeping the twist gentle.
2. Maintain an upright spine to prevent strain on your back.
3. Ensure your front knee doesn't extend beyond your ankle to maintain balance.
4. Remember to breathe deeply to enhance relaxation and flexibility.
5. Avoid excessive arching by engaging your core and tucking your tailbone slightly.

Chair Revolved Boat Pose

Chair Revolved Boat Pose is a yoga asana that combines elements of two different poses: Chair Pose (Utkatasana) and Revolved Boat Pose (Parivrtta Navasana).

INSTRUCTION

1. it toward the front edge of the chair, feet flat on the floor.
2. Lean back slightly, engage your core, and lift your feet off the ground.
3. Extend your arms forward alongside your legs.
4. Twist your torso to the right, bringing your left hand to the outside of the right knee and your right hand behind you.
5. Hold for a few breaths, then switch sides.

MISTAKES TO AVOID

1. Ensure your core muscles are engaged to maintain balance and stability.
2. Keep your spine straight to avoid hunching forward, which can strain your back.
3. Lift your chest and open your shoulders to avoid rounding your upper back.
4. Keep both legs lifted and engaged to maintain the pose's integrity and effectiveness.

Chair Revolved Side Angle Pose

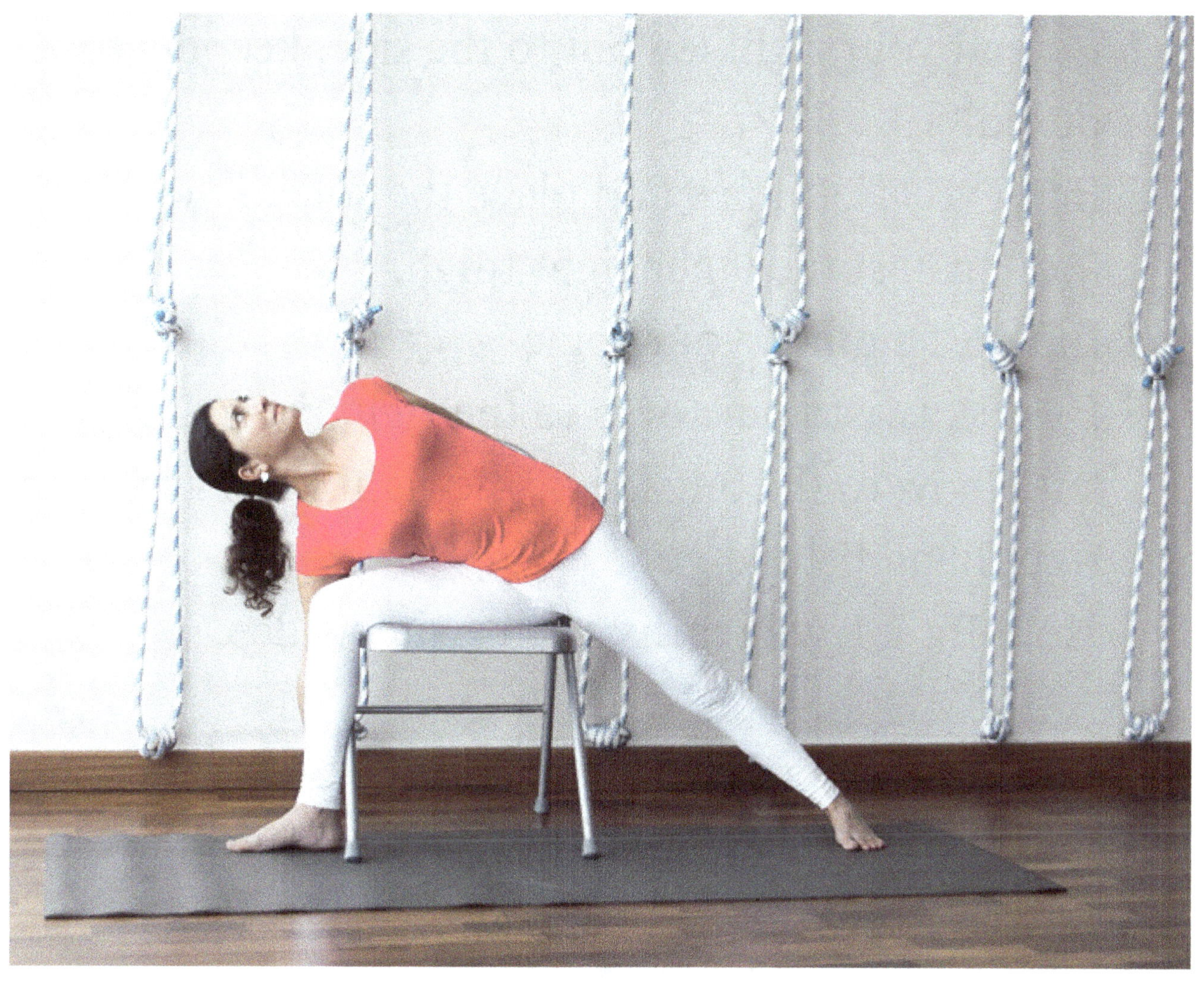

The Chair Revolved Side Angle Pose is a yoga asana (pose) that combines elements of Chair Pose (Utkatasana) and Revolved Side Angle Pose (Parivrtta Parsvakonasana). It's a variation that challenges balance, strength, and flexibility while engaging multiple muscle groups and promoting spinal rotation and elongation.

INSTRUCTION

1. Sit tall with feet flat on the floor.
2. Extend your right leg out to the side, keeping foot flexed.
3. Bend your left knee and place the sole of your left foot against the inner right thigh.
4. Inhale, lengthen your spine.
5. Exhale, twist your torso to the right, bringing your left elbow to the outside of the right knee and your right hand behind you.
6. Hold for a few breaths, then switch sides.

MISTAKES TO AVOID

1. Keep your spine straight to prevent slouching.
2. Ensure your feet are firmly planted to avoid wobbling.
3. Relax your shoulders and keep them away from your ears to prevent tension.
4. Rotate from your waist, not just your shoulders, to avoid strain.
5. Ensure your bent knee stays directly over your ankle to prevent injury.

28-DAY CHALLENGE

Week 1: Foundation and Awareness

- Day 1-7: Begin with basic seated postures and focus on breath awareness. Spend 10 minutes daily cultivating mindfulness and grounding.

Week 2: Mobility and Gentle Movement

- Day 8-14: Introduce gentle movements to mobilize joints. Explore neck, shoulder, and spine movements while seated. Gradually increase session duration to 15 minutes.

Week 3: Strengthening and Balance

- Day 15-21: Incorporate chair-based strength exercises. Engage core muscles and work on seated balance poses. Aim for 20 minutes daily.

Week 4: Mindful Flow and Relaxation

- Day 22-28: Combine learned movements into a flowing sequence. Emphasize breath synchronization. End each session with a guided relaxation or meditation. Aim for 25 minutes daily.

28-DAY CHALLENGE

Daily Tips:

- Stay Consistent: Commit to the challenge daily, even if it's a short session.
- Mindful Eating: Pair chair yoga with mindful eating practices for holistic well-being.
- Listen to Your Body: Modify poses as needed and avoid pushing yourself too hard.
- Journaling: Record your experiences, noting any changes in mood, energy, or body awareness.
- Celebrate Progress: Acknowledge improvements in flexibility, balance, and overall well-being.

Weekly Fitness

Week _______________________

Month _______________________

Monday Exercises:

Tuesday Exercises:

Wednesday Exercises:

Thursday Exercises:

Friday Exercises:

Saturday Exercises:

Sunday Exercises:

Weekly Goals

- ☐ _______________________
- ☐ _______________________
- ☐ _______________________
- ☐ _______________________

My Motivation

Notes / Reminder

Weekly Fitness

Week _______________________

Month _______________________

Monday Exercises:

Tuesday Exercises:

Wednesday Exercises:

Thursday Exercises:

Friday Exercises:

Saturday Exercises:

Sunday Exercises:

Weekly Goals

- [ ] _______________________
- [ ] _______________________
- [ ] _______________________
- [ ] _______________________

My Motivation

Notes / Reminder

Weekly Fitness

Week _______________________

Month _______________________

Monday Exercises:

Tuesday Exercises:

Wednesday Exercises:

Thursday Exercises:

Friday Exercises:

Saturday Exercises:

Sunday Exercises:

Weekly Goals

- [ ] _______________________
- [ ] _______________________
- [ ] _______________________
- [ ] _______________________

My Motivation

Notes / Reminder

Weekly Fitness

Week _______________________   Month _______________________

Monday Exercises:

Tuesday Exercises:

Wednesday Exercises:

Thursday Exercises:

Friday Exercises:

Saturday Exercises:

Sunday Exercises:

Weekly Goals

- ⬤ ☐ _______________________
- ⬤ ☐ _______________________
- ⬤ ☐ _______________________
- ⬤ ☐ _______________________

My Motivation

Notes / Reminder

Weekly Fitness

Week _______________________

Month _______________________

Monday Exercises:

Tuesday Exercises:

Wednesday Exercises:

Thursday Exercises:

Friday Exercises:

Saturday Exercises:

Sunday Exercises:

Weekly Goals

- ☐ _______________________
- ☐ _______________________
- ☐ _______________________
- ☐ _______________________

My Motivation

Notes / Reminder

Weekly Fitness

Week _______________________   **Month** _______________________

Monday Exercises:

Tuesday Exercises:

Wednesday Exercises:

Thursday Exercises:

Friday Exercises:

Saturday Exercises:

Sunday Exercises:

Weekly Goals

- ⬤ ☐ _______________________
- ⬤ ☐ _______________________
- ⬤ ☐ _______________________
- ⬤ ☐ _______________________

My Motivation

Notes / Reminder

Weekly Fitness

Week _________________________

Month _________________________

Monday Exercises:

Tuesday Exercises:

Wednesday Exercises:

Thursday Exercises:

Friday Exercises:

Saturday Exercises:

Sunday Exercises:

Weekly Goals

- ☐ _________________________
- ☐ _________________________
- ☐ _________________________
- ☐ _________________________

My Motivation

Notes / Reminder

Weekly Fitness

Week _______________________

Month _______________________

Monday Exercises:

Tuesday Exercises:

Wednesday Exercises:

Thursday Exercises:

Friday Exercises:

Saturday Exercises:

Sunday Exercises:

Weekly Goals

My Motivation

Notes / Reminder

Weekly Fitness

Week ______________________

Month ______________________

Monday Exercises:

Tuesday Exercises:

Wednesday Exercises:

Thursday Exercises:

Friday Exercises:

Saturday Exercises:

Sunday Exercises:

Weekly Goals

- ☐ ______________________
- ☐ ______________________
- ☐ ______________________
- ☐ ______________________

My Motivation

Notes / Reminder

Weekly Fitness

Week ___________________ **Month** ___________________

Monday Exercises:

Tuesday Exercises:

Wednesday Exercises:

Thursday Exercises:

Friday Exercises:

Saturday Exercises:

Sunday Exercises:

Weekly Goals

- ☐ ___________________
- ☐ ___________________
- ☐ ___________________
- ☐ ___________________

My Motivation

Notes / Reminder